The BEST LIFE

THE KEY TO LIVING

STOP ENDLESS DIETING AND START LIVING AGAIN WITH A NEW CLARITY

Fourteen Health Experts Explain The Truths To Lasting Health and Expose The Myths That Prevent You From Success

The Best Life
The Key to Living

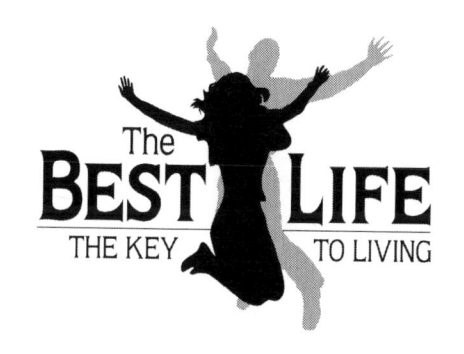

CONTRIBUTING AUTHORS:
SHALEENA ANAND
JULIE BALDERRAMA
KEITH COLBY
STEVE CONSIGLIO
ALEX DESROSIERS
STACIE DICKERSON
GINA FAUBERT
GINA FITZPATRICK
CAROL FROEHLICH
TRACY HAMMONS
ROSS JOHNSON
ALEXANDER KLAUS
MARK NIEMCHAK, DC
MARCOS SAYON

EDITED BY
ALEX CHANGHO & MICHAEL CUDDYER

The Best Life
THE KEY TO LIVING

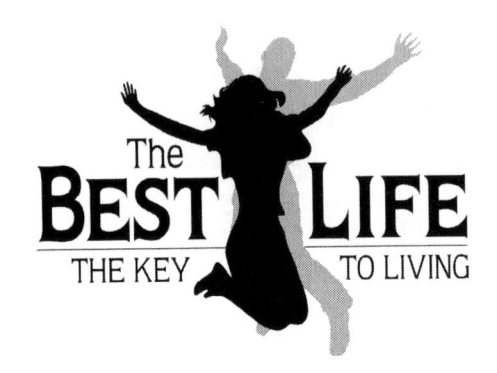

Copyright © 2016 Alex Changho

All Rights Reserved. No part of this publication may be reproduced in any form or by any means, including scanning, photocopying, or otherwise without prior written permission of the copyright holder.

THANK YOU

Thank you for purchasing this book.

It is our goal that more people are introduced to the concepts of true health and living The Best Life.

By purchasing this book and reading it, you will learn more about health and wellness, and find ways to make an impact in your own life.

In addition, 100% of the royalties of *The Best Life: The Key to Living* are being donated to the Anthony Robbins Foundation, which supports many initiatives that help youth, prisoners, and the homeless worldwide.

You're not just transforming your own life with this book, but helping the lives of others.

TABLE OF CONTENTS

Introduction – How to Use This Book - *Alex Changho* 1

Chapter 1: Waking Up – A Nutrition Journey – *Steve Consiglio* 7
Chapter 2: Living Longer & Healthier – *Carol Froehlich* 17
Chapter 3: Unhealthy Misconceptions – *Keith Colby* 29
Chapter 4: The Mindset of Weight Loss – *Alex Desrosiers* 39
Chapter 5: Neurofeedback & Your Best Life – *Gina Fitzpatrick* 51
Chapter 6: One Step At A Time – *Stacie Dickerson* 61
Chapter 7: Mindfulness & Meditation – *Shaleena Anand* 69
Chapter 8: The Eat Bacon Diet – *Mark Niemchak, D.C.* 81
Chapter 9: Fitness Failed Me – *Ross Johnson* 87
Chapter 10: Psychology in Fitness Training – *Marcos Sayon* 101
Chapter 11: Healthy Together – *Tracy Hammons* 109
Chapter 12: The Definition of True Health – *Gina Faubert* 119
Chapter 13: Qigong - Cultivating Life Energy – *Julie Balderrama* 133
Chapter 14: Health, Wealth, and Happiness – *Alexander Klaus* ... 145

Your Next Step: Decision and Action 157

Introduction: How to Use This Book

By Alex Changho
Cary, North Carolina

I'm not at all a health professional.

In fact, I'm far from it. During my adult life, I have bounced around from an eating plan to workout plan to this diet or that diet. And each had some sort of result. I read one book, I followed one fad, I saw some study on television and thought to myself, "That sounds smart, I'll do that."

Does any of this sound familiar to you?

If you're like me, and most people seem to be, this is not uncommon. We, as a public have access to so much information that it is hard to sift through it to see what works (and what doesn't). There are so many diet plans, weight loss programs, and fitness products out there that I ask myself, "Which one should I do?"

But there is definitely one thing that I know for certain: there is a difference between being fit and being healthy.

Early in my adult life, I was quite active and athletic. I ran a martial arts school, trained daily, was on the floor teaching 5 nights a week, and kept active almost all the time. I worked out, went to the gym, took supplements, and tried to bulk up.

I read the fitness magazines on how to get six-pack abs, bigger biceps, and tried to decipher how to look great naked.

As my business matured (as did I), my priorities shifted. I was getting great results, I attracted a wonderful woman, my clients loved me, and my fitness wasn't as important to me anymore. My waistline grew, but it didn't matter as much to me, because my concerns were external, how I looked on the outside. And as it mattered less and less to me, it took a toll on my health.

Then in March 2010, I attended a personal development seminar (as have a few of the authors in this book) that opened my eyes. I'll spare you the details, as I know that a few of the authors will talk about it later in the book. But I will stay this: I realized the importance of true health.

True health is what is vital to our lives. It is the foundation of our daily activities that leads us to live the best life.

What I thought was simply a matter of what you eat and what exercises you do turned out to be a much more holistic concern. Not just what I put in my mouth three times a day (or six, depending on the plan I was on at the moment), and what fancy exercise I was doing.

It was my environment. It was my stress. It was about the kinds of things I was putting into my body. It was the beliefs I had, the things I was saying to myself. It was even the way my brain was working.

No one talked about that in the men's fitness magazines with the half naked dude with a six-pack on the cover.

So I followed a path, like many of the authors in this book, of discovery, learning, and transformation. From what I did, I dropped 25 pounds of fat, and was more energetic.

Could I have researched this and figured it out from the Internet? Possibly. But by having a mentor, a structured plan to follow, and accountability, I was successful.

So here is what I have put together for you. Within these covers are the professional opinions of fourteen different experts in health. Some focus on psychology, others on nutrition. Some will talk about the importance of your environment.

There are differing opinions in this book. Some are wildly disparate! And guess what? It's okay. They all have results.

As there are seven billion people on this planet, there is more than one way to live the best life.

Here is what you can do:
1. Find a chapter that resonates with you. You might read this cover to cover, or more likely, you'll have met one of the authors and already been drawn to their message. Read that chapter and see how it fits with your life.
2. Feel free to read the other chapters, because there are different areas of focus, as well as different opinions. Learn about what fits for you.
3. Take action with the recommendations.

Living the best life does require that you do things differently in your life. So take steps in the direction you want to go.

BONUS: knowing myself, and maybe you're like this too, I have a tendency to play in my area of expertise. And as I opened this introduction, I am not by any means a health expert. I am knowledgeable, but I invest my time and energy into my areas of genius and impact on the world. So I choose to do one more thing, and you may want to consider this too:

If you resonate with a certain message, plan, or structure, then take action with it, and also go hire someone to help you get there. That's right, I'm telling you to go invest in a mentor in true health.

It might be the author of the chapter. If it's logistically difficult to hire them, find someone who can help you.

I have a personal trainer with whom I have worked for two years. I hire him to make sure I get my workouts in. This allows me to focus on my areas of impact (my business and my non-profit) while still doing the workouts that he instructs me to do, to have the foundation of energy I'm looking for.

By doing this, not only do I move towards living the best life for myself, but through my work, I can help others live their best life.

These fourteen experts are at your disposal. All the best to you!

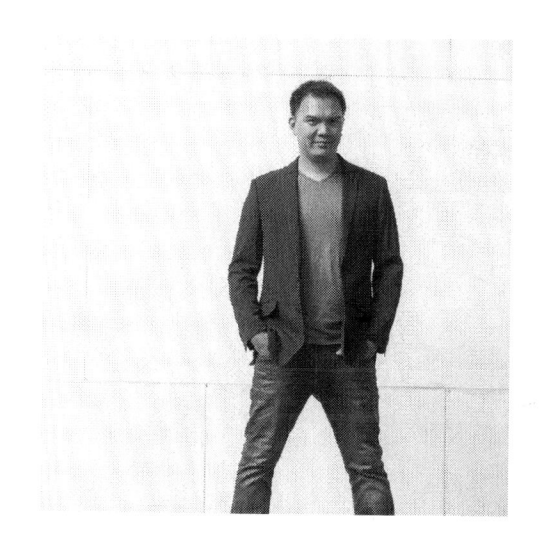

Alex Changho is a lifestyle and business coach. With almost two decades of experience leading and motivating others, and running a business, he helps business owners integrate their life's mission and career with their personal side of their life.

Alex is the founder of BULLYPROOF America, a non-profit with the mission of helping local communities educate families about bullying and help create confident kids.

An accomplished speaker and presenter, Alex is a Master NLP Practitioner and Trainer, Senior Leader with Anthony Robbins, and Master Strengths Coach.

Alex lives in North Carolina with his cat Bert.

For more information, visit www.alexchangho.com.

Chapter 1: Waking Up - A Nutrition Journey

By Steve Consiglio
Henrico, Virginia

I lost nearly a decade of my life—and almost lost my life entirely—to chronic fatigue.

The condition crept up on me over the course of ten years. It started off nearly unnoticeable—some illnesses here and there, an increased need for naps, sleepiness while working or driving, and difficulty getting off the couch (not due to injury, mind you—it was pure lack of desire). In the mornings, I was irritable, but I told myself that was normal. No one *really* likes to wake up, right? Then, it got worse. I had chronic fatigue: devastating exhaustion hit me, like clockwork, at 3PM each day. I was a personal trainer at the time, and I'd catch myself falling asleep, standing up, as I was training clients. This was a daily occurrence.

Later, when I took a job as a financial consultant, I would pass out cold on my desk in the middle of a case. Out of desperation, whenever I had a spare 15 or 20 minutes, I would close my door and lay down on a yoga mat for a power nap.

I knew things were bad... but I didn't know how bad until one day, I dozed off while driving on the interstate. When I jolted awake, my car was sailing around a sharp curve with a drop-off just beyond it.

Talk about a wake-up call.

Moving Forward

When you're young, you think that looking good and being physically fit are the ultimate signs of good health. I was a very lean, skinny child and teenager, so I was always trying to bulk up by eating a lot of calories and exercising. Up until my early twenties, I thought I was healthy. That is when my energy levels plummeted for seemingly no reason.

I may have been lean and muscular, but my body wasn't supporting true cellular health. The outside looked fine, but inside, physiologically, something was going wrong. Apparently being fit was not the be-all-end-all of true health.

After nearly a decade of suffering, I spent two nights at a sleeping clinic hooked up to electrodes. The doctor started asking me if I ever felt sad, and if I found that my low energy ever corresponded to low emotions. Of course, if you don't have the energy to do the things you normally enjoy—the things that make you feel productive and accomplished—it can certainly affect your self-esteem and mood.

The doctor concluded that I needed to be put on an antidepressant. Much as I respected his expertise and his opinion, I firmly declined. I knew myself well enough to know that I wasn't depressed, even if I was showing some of the symptoms of it, and that an antidepressant wasn't the right fit for me. Unfortunately, this left me back at square one, with no answers to my questions and no solution to my problem.

Luckily, I attended a seminar shortly afterward, not knowing that it would change my life. When the speaker started talking about vital health and energy, I immediately pulled out a pad and pencil, determined to listen and take as many notes as possible.

I listened to Tony Robbins talk about the Living Health principles—foods to avoid, controlled breathing, hydration, mindfulness, and other holistic solutions to energy issues. I learned that my high-calorie diet from high school and college (sometimes up to 6,000 calories a day) may have been harming by digestive system even if it wasn't showing up as body fat. The constant eating meant my body was always working overtime to digest the food, exhausting me in the process. The chronic fatigue was a symptom, and I had discovered the culprit.

The Art and Science of Food Combination

One of the best things I ever did was teach myself how to eat smarter instead of eating in excess. I adhered to a simple food-combining chart, which guided me on which foods to eat together, and which foods to eat separately.

Don't get me wrong. I'm certainly not a chemist or nutritionist, and to this day, my philosophy around health— specifically nutrition— is that everyone's body is different, and you should stick to the things that work for you. There are so many different philosophies and beliefs in terms of what you should and shouldn't eat, but the following information specifically made such a profound difference in my life that I chose to stick with it:

In any traditional American meal, you can usually find a carbohydrate and a protein—steak and potatoes, chicken and rice, hotdog in a bun, ham and biscuits, etc. They go together like... well, peanut butter and jelly (and bread)!

What I didn't know was that this type of diet forces the stomach to work against itself. When you consume proteins (eggs, dairy, avocado, nuts, seeds, soy, etc), your body releases one type of enzyme to help metabolize them. When you consume carbs (potatoes, pasta, lentils, grains, cereals, rice, etc), your body consumes another kind of enzyme to break them down. So when you eat them together, those enzymes are working hard against one another. This is exhausting for your digestive system, and therefore, for you.

So we don't want to have carbohydrates in the same meal as proteins, but they should both be eaten with non-starchy vegetables like spinach, zucchini, watercress, cabbage, celery, asparagus, cucumber, etc.

If you're going to consume fats and oils, those are better combined with carbohydrates rather than proteins. Fruits should be consumed on an empty stomach, not with other foods and especially not with a meal, which may cause fermentation on top of the other things you've eaten.

I also made some decisions about which foods I wanted to eat, and which foods I wanted to stay away from. I am not an advocate of refined white carbohydrates—white potatoes, cereals, white bread, white rice, etc—and anything you get in a box, like crackers and potato chips. All of these things are refined and get broken down into simple sugars in the body, so I like to steer more towards complex carbohydrates like quinoa, long-grain brown rice, breads made with sprouted grains, lentils, and sweet potatoes.

Like most people, I also used to drink fluids during meals, but this, too, prevents digestive enzymes from doing their jobs. Now, I try to stop drinking thirty minutes before a meal, and start again ten to thirty minutes afterward, to allow my stomach time to work on the food before having to process something else. If I feel thirsty in the middle of a meal, that's a pretty good indicator that the meal doesn't have enough water, which means it's probably not natural or healthy.

If this all seems complicated, a simple internet search for "food combination chart" yields a ton of great information. All of this became second-nature to me after many years of experimenting and practicing with my body and my personal health.

Bacteria and Dairy, Friends and Foes

I haven't been sick enough to require antibiotics since 2008, which was the year I started my morning ritual of taking a probiotic with a small bottle of water. This isn't a coincidence.

Our bodies need good bacteria, or "healthy gut flora," to boost the immune system and protect us from the bad stuff. We take PRObiotics to protect us from needing ANTIbiotics. Makes sense, right?

There are many types of probiotics, but in my opinion, any good bacteria contained in a probiotic that requires refrigeration probably wouldn't survive anyway once it enters your body. I choose probiotics with that patented Triosphere technology that is designed to protect it from shelf life and stomach acid, which means the healthy bacteria are actually released into your gut, and not killed upon impact. For me, this has worked for years to keep me healthy and antibiotic-free.

Of course when people think about probiotics, one of the first things they jump to is yogurt, but dairy is a complicated food group in of itself.

It's important to take any dietary concepts we've been conditioned to believe and examine them from scientific and common-sense standpoints. Humans are the only mammal that consume milk as adults even though we stop producing the milk-metabolizing enzyme at around age four, since we're not meant to have it once we're weaned. When you think about it this way, it's not surprising that so many of us experience mild or severe symptoms of lactose-intolerance.

My nighttime ritual used to be a glass of milk with a peanut butter and banana sandwich. I thought this was pretty healthy and ignored the stomachache I always got afterward. However, once I stopped consuming dairy, I found I was breathing easier, and my respiratory system was completely reinvigorated.

In the interest of full disclosure, I'm Italian, so I do enjoy a good slice of pizza, and after years of testing this theory I realized that—almost immediately after consuming a piece with cheese on it—my nose would begin clogging up, and the next day my chest would feel congested and uncomfortable.

So many kids these days are going through puberty too early. Girls are developing breast tissue at a young age, and a tragic number of our children in this country are obese. This isn't surprising when you consider that baby calves are meant to grow nearly a thousand pounds in a very short amount of time. Human children, of course, are not.

Why, then, do we insist on pumping them full of cow's milk? Ask any dairy company, and they'll answer, "Calcium!" So let's examine that.

Our bodies need to maintain a very specific pH balance to stay alive, and milk is very acidic. A high-acidity diet forces our bodies to try and correct the pH level, which it does by pulling alkalizing minerals from our bones. Over time, this actually weakens the skeletal system, causing osteoporosis and other conditions.

Yes, milk is high in calcium, but consuming milk to protect our bones is counterintuitive and makes them more brittle in the long run. Suffice it to say, dairy just doesn't do it for me anymore.

A Journey of the Body and Mind

Health is more than just nutrition and exercise—though I advocate being an active participant in both. The sooner we realize that protecting the mind is just as important as protecting the body, the better off we'll all be.

This "go, go, go" society we live in is so harmful to our bodies, especially at mealtimes. Is there any wonder our stomachs are struggling to digest things when we're in a constant state of high anxiety and high stress? Relax your mind before you eat. Your body will thank you.

The last eight years has been a time of trial and error for me, of experimenting and testing a number of theories, philosophies, and concepts. Once I found a system of nutrition that worked for me, I experienced a massive difference not just in my energy level, but my mental clarity and mood as well.

It's not normal to wake up cranky, exhausted, and in pain, and I was ecstatic to learn that I didn't have to anymore. How I handled stress changed; things just didn't seem to bother me as much as they used to. My temperament was more stable. I achieved joy, happiness, health, and stability, and there was no way I was going back. Maintaining these rituals—morning, meals, and night—has kept me on the right side of true health for eight years. Once I got to the other side of chronic fatigue and digestive distress, I realized... hey, I'm happy!

True health hinges greatly upon what goes on in a person's mind. The only thing we can control in this life is our thoughts, so lean toward happiness whenever you can. At any moment, we can choose to ask ourselves, "What do I appreciate right now? What in this situation can I be grateful for?" If there's one thing you can start doing right this second to take the next step towards true health, it's to make a conscious decision to see the good in a situation, rather than focusing on what's wrong. If you can change your thoughts, you can change anything.

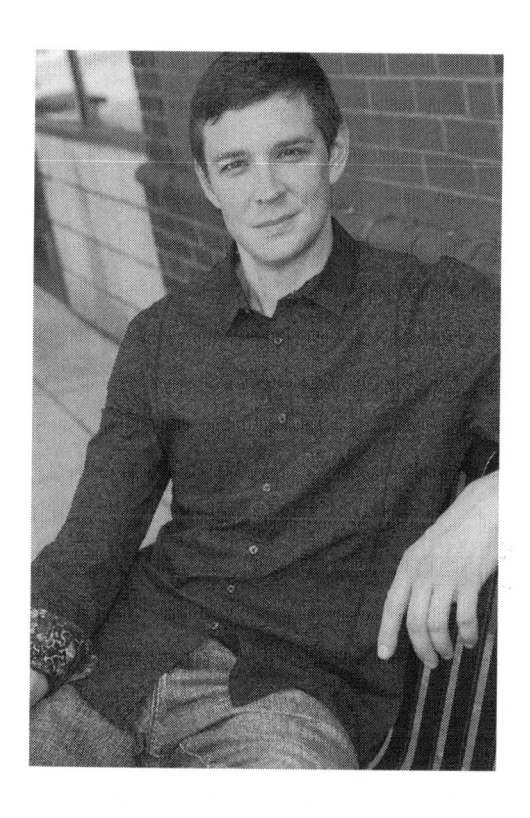

Steve Consiglio is an Investment Advisor Representative in Richmond, VA. He believes in not only providing a healthy financial lifestyle for his clients, but also in creating wealth in the body by utilizing his education and background in sports medicine and exercise science.

Steve helps his clients with psychology and a healthy mindset, personal achievement, nutrition, fitness, body work, as well as financial wealth accumulation and protection.

He obtained his B.S. degree from Roanoke College and a M.S. from Virginia Commonwealth University. He is a sought after speaker and a Master Practitioner in Neurostrategies and NLP.

Chapter 2: Living Longer & Healthier

By Carol Froehlich
New Rochelle, New York

Is it possible to live a longer, healthier, active life under the myriad of products that we are consuming and/or expose to on a daily basis? Is it possible to use products that are in harmony with nature and also be effective? These are questions that people are asking me all the time, and I am delighted to have this opportunity to share with you the powerful journey that brought about those answers into my life with such a clarity that my personal life and the life of my family was dramatically transformed.

My Story

My two beautiful children played every day while running in and out of my beautiful white, colonial house where I was living the

American "dream" in the suburbs with my British husband.

Since I had always liked having my own money, I started a small business from home as a children's entertainer. Since I was an opera singer and musical theater performer before having kids, entertaining little ones was a natural fit. Thus, I created a streamlined process for classes, events, and birthday parties that worked around my kids' schedule. I could even bring my kids with me to the events! Music Movement Tunes & Tales was a big happy success until my awful chronic allergies turned into adult asthma. It stopped me on my vocal, and energy, tracks. I could hardly breathe, let alone sing. Since my kids were only 3 and 6, and I had no help to care for them during the day, I didn't know what I was going to do next. My doctors had put me on asthma inhalers and prednisone (a very heavy duty prescription drug to reduce inflammation with huge side effects). I was one sick mama!

I searched for natural solutions, but in the pre-internet era that sort of information was hard to find. Finally, a friend suggested products she used and the results were miraculous! Six-and-a-half weeks later my allergies and asthma were gone. I tossed the prescription drugs right out, and I was over-the-moon about the products given that my health has been completely restored. Naturally, I became obsessed with these products. Quickly, my friends and family noticed the dramatic health difference in me, and not only wanted to know what I was using, they wanted to try it too. It was a natural transition to sell those products to other health-conscious people. And in just a few short months my little part-time hobby with this company made more money than the six years I spent in the children's entertainment business!! Thus, I retired "Music Movement Tunes & Tales."

Following my passion put me in a good place for life's next curveball. A few years later, after a very rocky marriage, my husband abandoned me on a month's notice. He left me and the kids with the unpaid bills, the mortgage, the taxes, the upkeep of the house, and more. Heck, the lease on the van was about to end too! So my little part-time hobby became a full time career from home that supported me and my kids. The income paid all the bills, earned me a new car, free vacations, and much more. That was 20 years ago.

I am inspired to share the valuable knowledge I have accumulated over a life time of personal health growth with anyone who is ready to receive and benefit from this life-saving information. If I can bring a third of the wellbeing my neighbor brought into my life and family by sharing this phenomenal knowledge with anyone, then my job is done; I am fulfilled. At first, I disregarded the information my neighbor was sharing for many months because I thought my over the counter vitamins were the ultimate solution to keep me healthy, until I realize they were not helping me at all. After I switched to these products, I started feeling better within days, and as a consequence, I started looking better. This cycle of betterment attracted fantastic events and people into my life. I further discovered that personal fulfillment is enhanced through the ability to make a difference in the lives of people beyond my family circle, and thus this chapter in this book was born.

What's Behind Most Product Labels?

Unknown, unsafe, unreliable
As a general rule, it is unknown, unreliable and unsafe what is behind most product's labels. Indeed, ninety (90%) of most goods found in our retail stores may not be as healthy as we think, and often people are not aware of that fact. Even though, there are good companies that offer healthy products; they can just be hard to find. The traditional "store experts", for example, are not interested in your health, they are interested in your money. When I walked into a retail store 20 years ago, and asked the "store expert" for the best supplements in the store, he referred

me to what most people use. That's the level of their expertise! They really don't know what is behind the label, and it is not their priority.

Governmental guidelines are very limited for the supplement and nutritional industry, and thus we have to create and strictly enforced our own guidelines to protect our health. However, be aware that even the most keen reader of the content on the labels would be lost when trying to identify a good supplement. Indeed, a very good friend of mine who is a nutritionist was taking a prenatal vitamin from a Whole Foods store thinking it was safe to do so, but it turned out to be unsafe. Low key governmental guideline allows for unsafe products.

Lack of guidelines have been the cause serious illness among consumers of Whole Foods products, and not because the Whole Foods stores are bad, but because Whole Foods does not manufacture all the products they sell. Whole Foods stores have to rely on the supplier guidelines on purity and follow those guidelines. Even more worrisome, several Whole Foods' processing plants have been the subject of serious governmental violations. Furthermore, Whole Foods stores had many recalls on some supplements, protein bars, protein drinks that they distribute on behalf of third party. The recall list of products was and still is surprisingly long every month, and it ranges from food products to nutritional supplements. (Please see website www.foodsafetynews.com for in depth information). These very questionable Whole Foods store's practices make their products unreliable.

Thus, we must become an informed consumer if we would like to live a longer, healthier life. We ought to seek for supplements and nutritional products that are safe, clinically proven and guaranteed.

Why Are So Many Products Pulled Off the Shelves?

Bottom line: they have made people sick.
As wellness brands increased their presence in retail stores, the FDA moved into curbing the distribution of these products. While dietary supplement manufacturers and distributors are not required to obtain approval from FDA before marketing dietary supplements, there are very limited FDA rules, a company marketing dietary supplements is responsible for 1) ensuring that the products it manufactures or distributes are safe, 2) that any claims made about the products are not false or misleading, and 3) that the products comply with the Federal Food, Drug, and Cosmetic Act and FDA regulations in all other respects. That is the extent of governmental guidelines for the wellness industry! And despite all of these words of protection used by the FDA, the truth is that pesticides, genetically modified organism (GMO), and artificial ingredients are often present in supplements. Indeed, some ingredients could be harboring bacteria, molds, and fungicides right from the farm, increasing the risk of complications, which makes people sick.

With no strict regulation on bacterial testing, companies are free to distribute these products without conducting such tests. This particular situation took place many years ago with the raw ingredient named: Ginseng whose crop proved to be contaminated with harmful bacteria. Instead of removing off the shelves all the related products many companies continued to keep selling the contaminated supplements. During the Ginseng incident, the company I use had tested all raw ingredients as part of their very own strict testing guidelines, and verified the presence of the microorganisms in their raw Ginseng material. My company immediately discontinued production for months in all products containing the Ginseng material.

The weight loss industry is a huge area of concern link to the safety of nutritional supplements and protein shakes because the population is looking for a quick fix. Thus, it is the perfect industry to create fast results with permanent health problems. Seems like a new fad, a fast miracle supplement or a diet pops up weekly. You know the ad reads like this: "Lose 30 lbs in 30 days. Lose weight while you sleep. Eat as much as you want and whatever you want and lose weight." Naturally, many weight loss products are subject of recalls because they are not created thinking on your health but are created to make money for the company and thinking on making you losing weight at any cost, including your health.

In my 20 year journey toward healthy living, I also opted out of gluten products, which resulted in weight loss and a healthier, more energetic body. And yet, some gluten-free cookies come with high sugar content and other ingredients. If you love organic food, check to make sure it's truly organic! Don't settle for a quick fix. Consider taking the longer, yet more sustainable route, that yields optimal health lasting a lifetime. My doctor told me I would need inhalers for the rest of my life, but I went a step further to conquer my illness on my terms.

Today, an average 65 year-old takes nearly 14 different prescription drugs. However I, at 60, am taking none. My 90 year young mother takes one medication that is a tiny dose of blood pressure medication, and remains my greatest motivation and testimonial, as she still drives her car, write stories, visit museums, make sculptures, takes yoga, and attend daily lectures, and she lives on her own! Now she is excited about her next 90 years!

This is exactly what you will get under the right coaching, and it's my passion to help you feel and look great, and live a long healthy and active life!

Do You Know What Is Under Your Sink?

After hearing about my health story, a neighbor came to me for advice. She and her family were suffering from chronic allergies. I completed a health assessment on her and her home and discovered many toxic cleaners that were triggering their condition. After several weeks following the supplement program I recommended which included eliminating toxins from their home and replacing them with safe products that I use, they got better. In fact, this family still is thanking me after 9 years!!!

Here is a very short list of the main harmful and toxic ingredients your cleaning and laundry products are made of:

- Volatile organic cleaning compounds
- Kerosene
- Phenol
- Cresol
- Lye
- Hydrochloric acid
- Sulfuric acid
- Sulfamic acid
- Petroleum distillates
- Ammonia
- Sodium hydroxide
- Butyl cellosolve
- Phosphoric acid
- Formaldehyde
- Morpholine

These ingredients are found in over the counter cleaning and laundry products which are filled with harmful, toxic ingredients that will deteriorate the health of you and your family in a very short period of time. Furthermore, there are studies that demonstrate a measurable relationship between chemical toxins and learning disabilities, allergies, respiratory issues, asthma, skin irritations among others.

Thus, we must become an informed consumer if we would like to live a longer, healthier life. We ought to seek for supplements and nutritional products that are safe, clinically proven and guaranteed.

How Do You Become An Informed Consumer?

Interrogating Manufacturers
In order to become an informed consumer, we must become informed about the production process of the product we would like to consume. When buying nutritional supplements and related products, call the 800 number and ask for relevant clinical studies the company has conducted on the specific product you are about to buy. Make sure that the company is not providing you with a general clinical study another company has completed. In my coaching sessions, I emphasize that buyers call the number on the bottle to inquire more about the scientific research conducted on the brands, as well as their manufacturing policy and find out 1) if the product and its ingredients are outsourced, 2) what type of quality testing is performed on each ingredient of the product, 3) request scientific proof that the product will deliver the results claimed to the customer. The production process determines how well the product serves the needs of the users. You could be taking a compound full of impurities, for example, due to poor processing procedures. If a company declines to give information, or admits a lack of information, that should trigger doubts on the quality of the brand. While most companies strive to provide high-quality products, cutting corners to improve their product margins may mean those products contain contaminated elements or lessor quality ingredients. Don't be afraid to ask questions!

Get educated by accessing the following website
Visit householdproducts.nlm.nih.gov/ingredients.htm
1. Go to the National Institutes of Health Household Products Database and find out what you have in your home.
2. Enter names of chemicals and see which brands contain them.
3. Look up Toxicity Information or Health Information for the chemical.

Take Action
- Properly dispose of harmful products
- Find safer choices with the company I discovered 20 years ago, who have been leaders in the Green movement for over 50 years Go to www.ABreathAwayGroup.com

Weight Loss
When it comes to weight loss, it's about getting healthy for the rest of your life, creating lifestyle changes that includes exercise, meditation, and a positive mental attitude.

Lasting success starts with a complete program that it is based on deliciously simple products, designed to burn fat, not muscle. A diet rich in Non GMO, plant based protein, organic greens and fruits. Additionally, a simple program that is easy to follow and fits into a busy lifestyle.

As a health coach, I experience and create for my clients a healthy way into more energy, better sleep, sharper mental clarity, weight loss, and a greater sense of well-being. No wonder I enjoy working with a plethora of raving clients that I have been serving as their health coach for over 20 years!!

TRANSFORMING THE PLANET

The Earth remains our largest respiratory system, whose sustainability is critical to healthy living. The topic attracts high levels of emotions, due to the fact that the bulk of our pollution comes from our own homes. It is a field where collective responsibility and effort is paramount to achieving a clean environment for us and our children. Over the last 20 years of my work, I have been a staunch supporter of a sustainable environment, and educated families on their role of preserving the natural aspects of the Earth. Every person and/or household has a part to play.

Adopting sustainable habits could be as simple as 1) changing your light bulb, 2) recycling plastic containers and bags to lowering your contributions to landfills, and 3) changing your cleaning products to Non-toxic products. Keeping your house green clean can be key to living a longer, healthier life for all of us.

Today, it is very simple to get what you want; I can guide you to helpful resources and help you design your healthiest life. Other than professional coaching, my company offers a broad range of products, with a team of passionate scientists who are keen to improve people's lives. We distribute green products across the country.

Regardless of the size of the company, conduct research on them via the internet, and get the personal assurance of that brand before you put the life of your family at risk. Some of the industry leaders who make "green" household products operate the bulk of their businesses with toxic chemicals. They maintain a small line of green products, which earns them positive publicity. They use the money received to fund the manufacture of harmful chemicals you unwittingly buy; killing the Earth on your behalf. Making a simple call will allow you to get the help you need in understanding the product that works for you while keeping your children safe and planet clean.

The choice is yours to live your best life.

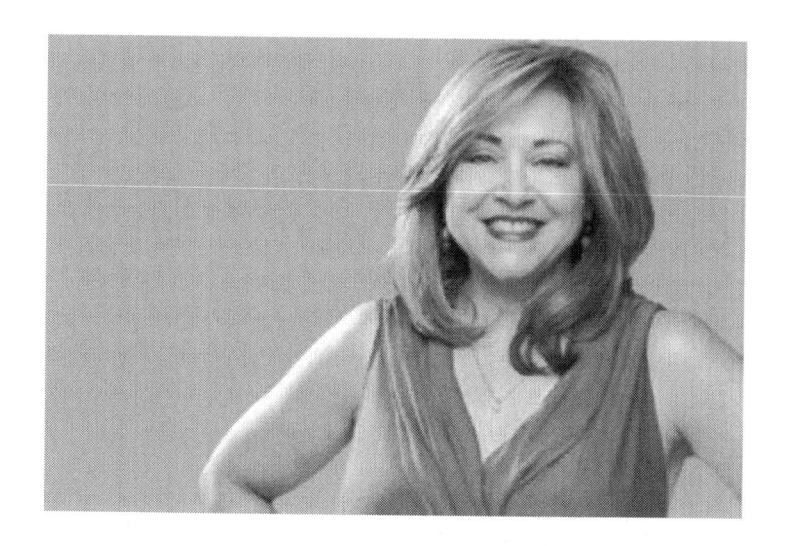

Since 1995 when green was a color, Carol has been coaching people across the country, and has been helping families get healthy and businesses go "green" with cleaning product needs. In addition Carol is certified and trained in the following areas:

- Health Life and Career Coaching
- Indoor Air Certification
- Neuro- Linquistic Programing (NLP)
- Leadership - 11 years with Anthony Robbins International
- Mastery University
- Business Mastery
- Leadership Bootcamp
- Crew Leadership
- High Performance Forum with Darren Hardy
- Progressive Workshop with Dr. Joe Dispensa

Carol's premier Health and Wellness products of choice is Shaklee Corporation and she has been a distributor since 1995. It is the Shaklee products that helped her get well. Her web site is: www.ABreathAwayGroup.com

She has accumulated her health knowledge through seminars with some the top scientists in the world on health.

Singing & performing for over 40 years, Carol studied and trained at Syracuse University, Indiana University, The Julliard School, and the American Institute of Musical Studies, in Graz, Austria. She studied theater at (HB Studio) The Herbert Berghof Studio, NYC. Is a member of Actors Equity for 4 decades and has performed musical theater and opera throughout the country and internationally. She believes movement is very important with health and she is an avid cycler, passionate about her Zumba and tennis.

She has performed at corporate events across the country at several major arenas, from the Breakstone Arena in Nashville Tennessee,to the MGM Grand Hotel Arena in Las Vegas, Nevada, The Cleveland Auditorium, Lincoln Center at Avery Fisher Hall and on the Red Carpet at the 2015 Oscars to name a few. She continues to inspire people through song and inspirational speaking and available for events.

To get your free personal health assessment go to: https://cfh.myshaklee.com/us/en/healthprint, or contact Carol at (914) 834-3137.

Chapter 3: Unhealthy Misconceptions

By Keith Colby
Brookline, Massachusetts

I've been a health researcher and coach long enough to notice some trends in my work. I'm approached over and over again with many of the same difficult obstacles standing between my clients and optimal health: weight loss, injury, pain, mobility issues, etc. Some want to train hard for a competitive sport and others just want to have an easier time partaking in fun activities again. I've met with older people who want to go on vacation, or go swimming, or go hiking, or just be flexible and strong enough to participate wholly in their lives without fear of injury. I've met with people who are not taking the time to care for themselves because they pay so much attention to others, and usually these individuals don't notice their own declining health until the problems can't be ignored any longer.

I've seen a variety of different people of all ages, from all walks of life, with issues that range all the way across the broad spectrum of health and wellness. Most of these challenges have one thing in common: they are hiding one or more sneaky misconceptions that need to be corrected before true progress can begin.

There are a lot of people out there—even health coaches and fitness instructors—who look good on the outside. That's what most people want, after all. We're chasing "The Look," the number on the scales, and all those cultural obsessions that leave us totally oblivious to the real needs of our bodies. Many of us have deduced that the way to get healthy is to train hard, eat lots of chicken and rice, take fish oil and weight proteins, avoid sugar, and work ourselves to the point of exhaustion. That's the way to strength and happiness, right?

The dirty secret is that, more often than not, those good-looking people can't sleep. They have cold hands and feet. They don't have a daily bowel movement. They may look ripped on the outside but are suffering on the inside. They may even have skin issues.

So if the people exerting hours of daily effort and thousands of dollars for wellness aren't truly healthy, does the average person stand a chance?

If you grew up chubby and slow like I did, you know that fierce exercise *seems* like the solution to all your problems. In my twenties, I exhausted myself with workouts. I trained as long as I could, got my heart rate up, lifted hard, and always pushed myself further than I did the day before. There was a time in my life where I was training six or seven times a week. I was big and strong, and doing everything I thought was required to be healthy and happy.

During that time, I also had acne so bad that I had to wear baseball caps in public. I went to clubs and drank a lot on the weekends. I fell into depression and took SSRIs. Looking back, I can see that exercise was <u>not</u> the solution to all of my problems. It was just a cover for anxiety, nervousness, and other feelings I couldn't control.

The most unfortunate thing about this part of my life was that I was actively promoting myself as a fitness trainer and a health expert. Had I known then what I know now—had I been able to read the following pages in my twenties—I could've done much better for my clients, and for myself.

Too many people today think about true health as simply the absence of disease—that if you're not sick, you're healthy. But disease is a destination, and a person who seems healthy might be unknowingly riding in the fast lane toward it.

Symptoms that are easy to dismiss as "stress" are always worth examining further. Exhaustion, joint pain, hair loss, moodiness, and a lowered immune system may not seem related, but they are certainly not conducive to a healthy lifestyle, and they may even be the precursors to something serious. A particularly nasty barrier for older people is the temptation to resign themselves to these and other hardships simply because they're told it's unavoidable. They may complain about pain and follow it with the phrase, "But I'm not as young as I used to be. This is normal." It doesn't have to be.

The definition of true health is so much simpler than many people realize. It's the ability to adapt to your environment and participate in your life as long as you can—a state of optimal, physical, mental, and social wellbeing. That is a goal achievable by anyone, at any time in their lives, and starting that journey may be as easy as debunking some pesky and dangerous myths about what it means to be truly healthy.

Movement is Life

Many of us spend a lot of time thinking about how to improve the quality of our workouts. We want to build as much muscle and burn as many calories as we can in the shortest amount of time. But what about improving the quality of our movement? Are exercise and movement essentially the same thing?

One of my mentors once told me, "Movement is mandatory. Exercise is optional." Our very survival depends on movement, and our bodies are designed to move and flow. We do not need to exercise to live.

But of course, the two concepts aren't entirely unrelated. Good exercise starts with healthy movement.

I was at a seminar in Boston when all of us were asked to break out and start doing a number of different activities to test our movement—the agility ladder, drills, etc. At the time, I was a big, muscular guy who could bench-press a lot of weight. I thought I was Mr. Strong and could do anything I wanted and look good at the same time. But these exercises completely whipped me. I couldn't move at all! From that day forward, my mindset shifted. I went from being concerned about exercise to being concerned about movement.

Spend a minute thinking about your last workout. Did you get equal contribution from all the joints in your body? Were certain joints taking on more stress than they should have? Do you think you were being efficient with your movements? Were you truly *feeling* the motions as they moved through you? Did you notice balance and steadiness in your feet? Were your muscles relaxed, or too tense? Could your joints move without restriction? Did certain movements force you past your threshold?

These questions should also be asked for activities outside of structured workouts. Your quest for healthy movement can start as soon as you wake up in the morning. How are you moving through your home, through your workplace, through the grocery store? How are you moving in your sleep? How are you holding yourself when you sit and stand? How are you interacting with your family? How are you taking out the trash?

Movement is life. Understanding that is the key to feeling better not just in your body, but in your mind; there are a multitude of complex ways in which two interact with and inform one another. When I see someone with a tight shoulder, I immediately look for where the tension is held in their bodies. Releasing that tension relaxes the mind, and a relaxed mind relaxes the entire body. The correlation is that powerful.

Understanding your body's movement is a lifelong process. Years of working out and exercise didn't prepare me for some of the movements I had to learn to participate in that seminar, or to begin studying internal martial arts. I was blown away by how difficult it was, how uncomfortable and out-of-shape I felt. My current master uses me as an example to the new students: "His chicken-step is good, but when he first started, he was shaking and sweating!" It's true. I may have been good at exercising, but learning to move appropriately in martial arts was one of the hardest things I've ever done.

The most important thing to know is that the movement and looseness of your body will affect the entire spectrum of your well-being. The quality of your movement can improve the quality of your workouts, your flexibility, the ability to utilize your strength, the quality of your sleep, and—odd as it may sound—even the quality of your interpersonal relationships. When the body can adapt to difficult situations, the mind will follow.

A Word About Sugar

What I knew about sugar in 2010 was what most people know about it today: it's toxic, it causes cancer, it's bad for you, and it's impossible to be healthy if you eat it. I was eating a lot of raw veggies at the time and staying away from meat so I could get my protein from other sources. I brought a big salad to work every day—beans, cauliflower, broccoli, etc. And, of course, I was avoiding sugar.

But even with that much-acclaimed "super healthy" diet, I didn't feel great. I had terrible gas, bad digestion, allergies, and no energy. I couldn't even get a good night's sleep. I knew I had to be missing something.

How do we reconcile sugar's bad rap with the fact that it's the body and brain's primary source of energy? The thyroid needs sugar to convert hormones. It helps our liver detoxify blood. It helps maintain muscle tissue. It increases metabolism. Sugar lowers stress hormones. It helps digestion. It can heal wounds. The list goes on and on. For those who partake, sugar can even help detoxify alcohol (some say) 80% quicker.

It's worth throwing out everything you think you know about sugar and rebuilding your knowledge base from scratch with well-rounded research. Many of us are simply confused about the many things sugar can do to *help* our bodies. Let's look at one of those things in particular:

Something that anyone can do to in their journey toward true health is improve the quality of their sleep—and that doesn't just mean just increasing the number of hours you spend in bed. Many people don't realize that truly restful sleep comes from increasing the body's metabolism through smart nourishment.

Stress hormones can run very high at night, a time when many of us sit and replay all the difficult interactions we had that day, beat ourselves up for all the things we didn't accomplish, and dread all the things that face us in the morning. We need a powerful friend in our corner to fight against all of that adrenaline and cortisol. Believe it or not, sugar (coupled with some fat) will give you that strong one-two punch you need to rest easy.

Many people are surprised about my personal secret for getting high-quality sleep: a small serving of clean ice cream, with no additives that will inflame the gut and intestines. Häagen-Dazs is my preferred brand.

Like everything food-related, sugar has its pros and cons. There's no question about that. But if having little bit of fat and sugar before bedtime improves the quality of your sleep, like it does mine, I can promise it'll be worth the extra calories.

Using Knowledge to Overcome Challenges

Fallacies and misconceptions get the better of the best of us. Even experts aren't immune to them. We learn more every day about what makes our bodies tick, and what makes them tick better. Together, we can use that knowledge to overcome many of the obstacles standing between us and our peak wellness.

I used to lecture to people about healthy living until the cows came home: "You need to do this. You need to stop eating polyunsaturated fats. You need to move more. You need to check your body temperature. You need to check your pulse." But that just wasn't effective for many people. I didn't like sounding like too much of an authority. I didn't like handing out "to-do" and "to-don't" lists.

Don't get me wrong; if a client asks me, "What should I eat? What should I do?" I will always work with them to discover good, customized options that work for them. But these days, I prefer to just share my story with people. I ask questions and give people books and articles to read for themselves so they can see what jumps out at them. Even though everybody (and every body) is different, it always helps to hear how others who have experienced a similar problem have solved it.

I also encourage people to take a good, honest look at themselves. Ask hard questions about your diet, your movements, your habits, that will allow yourself to see deeper into your own experience. Personal insight is so powerful, and many people will never take that first step forward until they truly see the issues for themselves.

The good news? You're probably not as bad off as you think you are. You're not broken. You're resilient, and you're doing okay. Look past the misconceptions and towards the things that will lead you down the road to true health. That's where your power is.

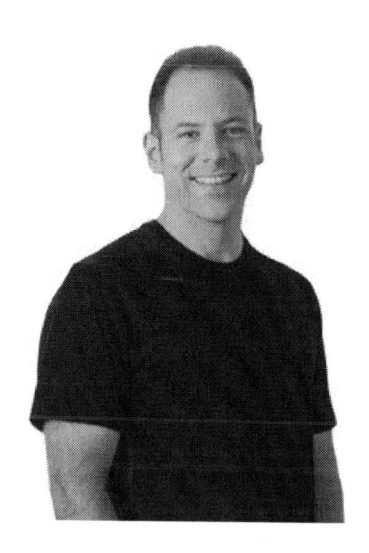

Keith Colby is a movement monkey, energy ninja, strength and health expert who has been in the health and fitness industry since 1996. Keith is known for being an information hound and prides himself on his unconventional methods that support a high running metabolism, health, longevity, pain relief, physiological and physical body function.

Keith has committed his life to seeking out the truths to health, longevity, and having a high metabolism. His own personal journey and experience has become the foundation of his teachings and has helped him better understand why sustainable health is not found through quick fix dieting, 90 days to fitness programs, 21 day weight loss programs, and over-exercising. But instead by increasing metabolism through the right nourishment, movement and strength, exercising less, getting enough rest and sleep.

Through his ongoing and always evolving research, reading, and personal experiences Keith has discovered that a high running metabolism combined with an understanding of where the human experience comes from is the basic foundation to health and well being. As an author, mentor, and teacher he coaches people from all walks of life on how to improve their health through fuel and nourishment, mind and thinking, movement and strength, rest and sleep.

Keith holds a degree in exercise science, is a Fellow of Applied Functional Science with the prestigious Gray Institute, Certified Strength and Conditioning Specialist, Certified Personal Trainer, was voted one of "America's Top 100 Personal Trainers" by Mens Journal Magazine, won a readers choice award for "Best Fitness Instructor" and has been featured in the Boston Herald.

For more information, visit www.keithcolby.com.

Chapter 4: The Mindset of Weight Loss

By Alex Desrosiers
Ottawa, Canada

Today, excess weight is a health problem that draws attention from the medical community all across the globe. While the exact classification of obesity remains debatable, one thing that is well known are all the complications that being obese increase the risks of developing. The complications including cancers, diabetes, cardiovascular diseases and much more.

When I started thinking about helping individuals with excess weight, one element became clear to me very quickly. In order to offer individuals with a lasting solution for Permanent Weight Loss, it was a must to include Human Psychology along with nutrition and exercise. While the current emphasis in the Fitness Industry is on nutrition and exercise, it also became clear to me that a person's mindset was the element that either caused an individual to maintain the lost weight or to regain the weight they had just worked so hard to lose.

You have probably seen many enrolling in weight loss programs and failing to lose weight or regaining the weight back quickly after losing it. That makes complete sense with the focus of these weight loss programs being on the need to increase exercise and lower calorie intake per day. While these two elements seem like the magical formula, weight loss is actually a much more complex process for the large majority of individuals, which needs to contain human psychology. Failing to address the psychology behind weight loss will very often lead to individuals losing their motivation and stopping the program. It can also lead individuals to regain the weight as soon as they have finished the program because they failed to make the mental shifts required to keep the weight off. Anyone wishing to have a lasting solution for weight loss needs to understand some specific distinctions about the psychology behind it.

Current Trends

There is a growing hype on different media outlets and social media on success stories from people that have successfully lost weight. Also, the media publish more and more about scientific studies results on the topic of weight loss. The problem with the studies being published in media is that the studies' conclusions get taken by the reader as the new "truth". One study which was recently published suggests that after individuals lost substantial amount of weight, their bodies and their metabolisms retaliated to regain the lost weight. Having completed a Masters in Epidemiology, I can say without any doubt, that for a conclusion like the one suggested in that study to be accepted, several more studies need to be made to confirm these findings and with higher sample size (only 14 participants were studied here). However, like mentioned previously, the media coverage was so important that the conclusion gets accepted as the new "truth". One participant in the study lost 239 pounds in 7 months. It is not hard to realize that this man's body would abnormally react after this extreme weight loss. If sustainable weight loss methods had been used and that these participants would have been getting the chance to understand the psychology behind weight loss, I am convinced that they would have never regained the weight.

The Mind Factor

individuals came to me because they were tired of regaining back the weight they had worked so hard to lose. For many of them, they kept regaining the weight back for one reason. They had never changed their identity (or how they defined themselves with regards to body weight). Inside their minds, they still defined themselves as a "fat" person. This identity of being "fat" influenced their emotional states, which end up influencing their behaviors and ultimately end up influencing their results, which causes them to consistently return to the results consistent with how they define themselves ("I'm fat"). Self-Development giant Tony Robbins says the following "The strongest force in the human personality is our need to stay consistent with how we define ourselves." This is why a person that keeps defining themselves as "fat" will keep getting results that are consistent with a fat person.

Also, your health behaviors like what you eat and if you exercise or not, come from your thinking in your mind. Once an individual learns how their thinking influences their behaviors, which then influence their end results, it gives them the possibility to be self-reliant with their body weight for life.

Many of these individuals did not understand before why they kept regaining weight (not shifting their identity being one of the many possible reasons). The current weight loss industry gives people with excess weight incomplete solutions. For individuals to be able to lose weight and keep in off, it is essential that key distinctions about the psychology of weight loss be given to them, so that they can adopt a mindset, which will lead them to win and create a new healthy lifestyle.

The Formula For Shifting Your Thinking

When people change their actions consistently, their identity can end up falling into place. However, there is a much easier way to do this. The easiest way is to first help someone shift their thinking and identity to the ones of a person with a healthy body weight, which will end up generating behaviors and ultimately results that are congruent with a person with a healthy body weight. However, that does not happen within a day, week as it takes some time to condition in this new identity and thinking into their new lifestyle.

Many different strategies can be used to help a person make this shift and they will need to be tailored specifically to each person. Some individuals end up using excess weight to protect themselves against perceived threats. Others develop a weight problem as a way to deal with stress or negative emotions. So this is why it's crucial that the process be individualized.

The problem with traditional weight loss programs is that they don't realize that excess weight is often just a symptom and that without addressing the causes, it will keep showing up in the person's life.

Self-Awareness

When people come to me, most often show some level of self-awareness that it is the psychology rather than the nutrition and exercise that negatively influences their progress. Most are quite aware of the particular issues limiting their ability to shed off weight sustainably. They acknowledge the presence of some resistance to nutrition, exercise and keeping up with the programs. Current weight loss methods do not allow them to lose weight and maintain it as these programs don't address human psychology.

My Work Experience

I have helped many women that have encountered some unwanted attention due to their bodies in their teen and young adult lives. Most of them would turn heads because of their great physical appearance. For some of them, this unwanted attention from men triggered such pain and fear, that they made a decision (even if not always consciously). That decision was that by changing their physical appearance to one that is less attractive, either by putting on a lot of weight or losing a lot of weight to lose their feminine curves, so that they would no longer get the unwanted attention and therefore wouldn't be exposed to the fear or pain.

For others, it was something that someone said to them while they were a kid, like "you're so fat" and that they accepted that as the truth and adopted it as their real identity regarding body weight. Parents have such power of their kids because whatever a parent says is taken as the gold standard. Unfortunately, in some cases, it leads to kids adopting an identity that is very disempowering. While it could be the best intention to help the child take care of their health, I have helped women in their 50's that still had a disempowering identity that they adopted unconsciously at a much younger age because of such negative comments.

I have great respect for people that work in dietetics, personal trainers, and doctors in the field of weight loss. Unfortunately, it is clear to me that the whole weight loss field is missing a big part and that part is the effects of human psychology on weight loss.

Also, when addressing the psychology part, it can often lead to figure out causes that no diet, exercise program or pill will ever resolve.

If you fail to address the mental part, the vast majority of individuals will face mental barriers that will prevent them from either following through or from getting any lasting results. So my part is to help them get rid of the mental barriers, so they can continue on their weight loss path much more easily and get permanent weight loss results.

Success Stories

Since I started studying coaching, I have helped many women that were successful in all spheres of their lives, but just couldn't solve the body weight sphere, despite having tried all the different "solutions" available in the market. Whenever we look at their mental patterns, it becomes clear that they had limiting patterns that were preventing them from getting lasting results. Often when working on emotions, past conflicts and the mindset part, the person will start losing weight faster than they ever did with nutrition or exercises strategies. There is so much still to be understood about the incredible mind-body connection and how to harness it for getting the optimal results.

By not completing my medical training and the opportunity going to study Psychology and Neuro-Linguistic Programming, instead it gave me to appreciate the role of a person's psychology with relation to their health and body weight. Before I had that opportunity, anyone who would have tried to convince me that excess body weight has such a huge link to a person's mental patterns, I would have labeled as fraudulent and would have discouraged people to go seek such "mind-body methods" at any cost. It wasn't until I realized that all the medical, health and scientific knowledge that was regarded as the "ultimate truth" was actually just a very important part of a much bigger picture.

Myths About Weight Loss

The entire concept of tracking your calories is not as easy as it sounds and even the concept of calorie counting itself has some pitfalls. It is easy to say that someone needs 100g of protein, but that person might end up absorbing just a part of it. So many factors end up influencing what truly happens in a person's body, that while calorie tracking and counting can be useful, it has to be used very carefully. It can actually have some negative consequences like in the following example. A person is given a diet that is based on severe calorie restriction and might have a daily target of 1200 calories. However, often individuals who track calories will want to make that they are not getting more than 1200 calories, so they end up eating less than the amount of calories prescribed. In addition to this, remember that all the calories eaten are not necessarily absorbed. So this person could have been given a diet with already extreme caloric restriction for maximum fat loss, but now they actually are getting a lot less than 1200 calories and can end up going into "fat accumulation mode" because they did not get enough calories. So what was intended to give maximum fat loss results, actually doesn't give any fat loss at all, but in that case actually results in fat gain. So this is why calorie tracking and counting has to be applied carefully especially in the case of severe caloric restrictions.

Another common pitfall is generalizing for the whole population. How often do we hear that we need to drink 8 glasses of water per day? While this might be true for a person with healthy body weight, it doesn't make sense to apply the exact same amount to someone that might weigh 100 pounds more because that heavier person will likely end up being dehydrated. Hydration being one key factor for optimal weight loss to occur. Adapting recommendations specifically for each person is crucial.

Here is another example of how generalizing can lead to unwanted results. One of the key concepts of weight loss is said to be to increase our level of physical activity. While this might be very useful for someone who is very inactive, for a person that is already very active trying to lose weight and that now would go and increase even more their level of physical activity working out 6 to 7 days a week, in addition to daily stressors, it might lead the person to accumulate high levels of cortisol that trigger fat accumulation instead of the initial weight loss intent. It is crucial for the body to have a balance between rest and demands on the body (workouts, daily stressors, work stressors, etc.) for optimal fat loss to occur.

Many people that came to seek my help were working out intensely 6 to 7 days a week with either no progress or gaining fat and living lives full of stressors. They are often left speechless when they start working out 3 days a week for 45 minutes to my suggestion and start losing weight, while they were getting no results on a 6 to 7 days/week schedule. The weight loss results come because the body is allowed to have sufficient time to recuperate and is no longer overwhelmed by the stressors.

The Diet Mindset

You have probably heard people say they are going on a diet to cut off some pounds. However, most of these diets are unhealthy and unsustainable making it hard to keep up until the end. When people fail to complete a given plan, a feeling of self-defeat sets in, making one accept the fate that they will never succeed in the endeavor. Some will start eating more healthy and exercising but after losing weight, go back to the old habits only to see the results reverse. They are likely to get into another diet to lose weight creating a cycle that is hard to break without dealing with the mindset and developing awareness. It calls for a permanent lifestyle change as opposed doing a diet for "x" amount of time. Unfortunately, many will be told that this is the only way to go to lose weight.

The first thing that I clarify with the individuals which I help is that there is no a diet or exercise system that will give them permanent weight loss results unless they also incorporate human psychology.

The biggest lie that you might have heard is that there is only one way to lose weight. This couldn't be further from the truth. In Neuro-Linguistic Programming, the Law of Requisite Variety states that people with the highest flexibility in a system win. People must understand that there are many ways to lose weight and that many different approaches can work. To get permanent results, it is critical to consider the psychology aspect of weight loss.

My Personal Experience

One of the motivational factors for helping individuals who are obese comes from personal experience of being clinically obese. Measuring 6'2" and with broad shoulders I could hide the weight more easily. I was what we call "skinny-fat". Which means a person which has high levels of body fat and very little muscle mass. I have now developed a very high muscle mass (comparable to professional athletes) and a body that is healthy. For lasting results, it wasn't until I truly began understanding the psychology behind weight loss that I was able to keep my body how I want it to look.

When I started losing weight, I only knew of one strategy to do so. I would get anxious to get injured and that I couldn't continue losing weight. It is only when I realized that there are many ways to lose weight and gained a lot of flexibility that I truly became the master of my body.

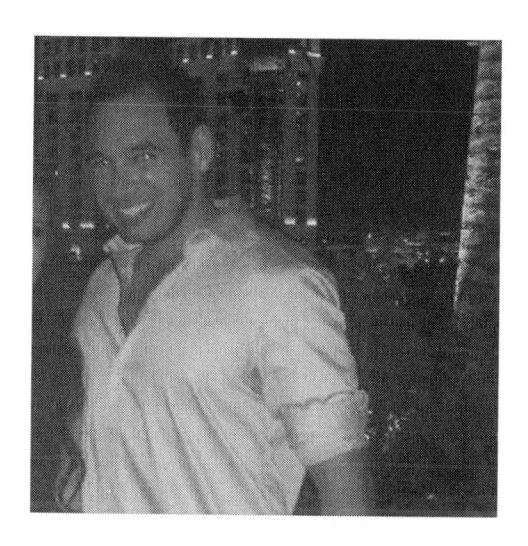

Alex Desrosiers B.Sc., M.Sc., (AlexDMindStrategist) focuses on Psychology and Neurosciences Coaching Specializing in Mind-Based Permanent Weight Loss for Obese and Overweight Women (who either can't seem to lose weight or can't seem to keep it off once they have lost the weight.)

Alex uses the knowledge and skills acquired during his extensive University Studies in the field of Medicine, Health Sciences and Public Health to have a unique perspective of the Human Body, Human Mind and Weight Loss.

Alex is also a Master NeuroStrategist and Master NLP Practionner from NeuroStrategies International lead by International Leader Steve Linder. This training enables Alex to understand in-depth Psychology and Neurosciences Applications and help individuals make lasting transformation in short periods of time.

For more information, visit www.alexdmindstrategist.com.

Chapter 5: Neurofeedback and Your Best Life

By Gina Fitzpatrick
Fort Lauderdale, Florida

The most impressive picture of a "best life" can be made by our think tank: the brain. It's not always easy to understand how our brain works, and how it can help us achieve our goals; luckily, there are people who specialize in that very concept, called "neurofeedback." These days, we're helping a variety of people all the time. From West Palm Beach down to Miami, Brain Training for You, continues to serve many on their journey towards vitality and wellness in order to experience their best life.

Neurofeedback, the Definition

In order to understand neurofeedback we must first know that our bodies contain more information and communications than the

World Wide Web. Each and every organ, muscle, bodily system and cell is talking and listening to one another. Keeping the lines of communication open would seemingly be important if we were to remain healthy.

Neurofeedback uses an electroencephalogram, or EEG, to measure your brainwaves, then offers real-time feedback so your brain can adapt in the moment. This training helps you improve your brain's function.

Technology Was Miraculous

Technological advancements these days have helped me make so much progress in my life, and also in the lives of the people around me. Yet, like many others, I am skeptical of many new technologies, or technologies I don't yet fully understand. Before investing in this machine I was actually a Neurofeedback client first. After experiencing my life changing results, I was sold. Within a month I bought the machine and within a year I was leaving my very comfortable, corporate job to go help others through neurofeedback.

One of my favorite client stories is about a gentleman in his 40s who was waiting around for the world to end, so really had no reason to get off his mother's couch and seize the day. Let's call him 'Doomsday Prepper'. He was so entrenched in his views that it kept him from renewing his driver's license, renewing his car registration and getting a job. His mother, with whom he still lived, was concerned enough by his views and lifestyle that she went in search of help which led her to me. She'd unfailingly drive him 30 miles to and from my house for each visit.

After the third session the gentleman's brother from the other side of the US called me and said, "I'm so thankful for what you are doing for my brother that I'll pay for his next seven sessions myself." Little did I know that the mother and brother were discussing about how after the third session he had decided it may be a good time to get a job and set some goals for the future rather than waiting around for the world to end. They were more than thrilled. The gentleman's brother soon after bought the same neurofeedback machine and is now helping others as well.

Another one of my favorite client stories is about a gentleman in his late 60s who had experienced electric shock therapy. We'll call him 'Marlin'. As I scanned my client, I noticed only half of the normal number of brainwaves was active. For all intents and purposes, only half his brain seemed to be functioning normally. He had very odd sleeping habits, rarely left his home to socialize and hadn't felt emotions since the electric shock therapy.

By the fourth session, he was starting to feel emotions again and his sleep schedule started to correct itself. With regulated sleep, and new emotions he had a renewed joie de vivre. By week three he was getting out of his home, socializing and exercising. He picked back up his piano playing and lost 25 pounds. He is now looking for dates online. Even his friend noticed he's made more progress in eight months with me than he did with twenty other years of medication and therapy from different medical professionals. His friend is now a client of mine as well.

Neurofeedback Is Key

When Marlin began neurofeedback training, he started to have emotions and began socializing with the rest of the world; every day, he takes a step towards living his best life. But what does "best life" mean?

For me, the best life is the balance between the mind, the body, and the spirit. In 11 years of working on myself, I can still see myself as a work in progress. Realizing that mental health was a key element of my physical health and overall happiness, I decided to study how neurofeedback works, and apply it to myself. After a few sessions, I realized that I could develop the technique even more through pairing it with coaching.

My Health Challenges

I wasn't like most other kids. I didn't get to play outside like "normal" kids did, because I spent the majority of my childhood (ages 2-9) in an oxygen tent in the hospital. I didn't get to experience the vivid colors of parks and playgrounds; I mostly saw the drab white of the inside of hospitals. I was allergic to pretty much everything.

It seemed as if no one had any idea what was going on with me. My parents would bring me to get my scheduled allergy shots without knowing that my system was already overloaded. Inevitably, I would have an asthma attack, followed by a trip to the emergency room, shots of epinephrine, followed by bronchitis and pneumonia which kept me in the hospital in the sterile oxygen tent. When I finally was released from the hospital, we'd see the allergist, get shots and repeat the same insane cycle.

I grew tired of this cycle of get shots, get sick stay in the hospital, repeat; so I decided to research alternative solutions on my own. Once I began to better understand what was going on inside my body, my spirits started to rise as did my ambitions to find a better answer. Since this early age I've always sought out a solution. I wouldn't settle for the "you're going to have to live with it" mantra I got used to hearing from so many.

Oddly enough, I sought out neurofeedback when I was looking to find a solution for my motion sickness. I learned that astronauts use the technology to alleviate their motion sickness. I figured my motion sickness is bad, but it couldn't be astronaut-bad, right.

When I entered the neurofeedback provider's office he ran some assessments and asked me for how long I had been experiencing this severe PTSD. He was actually shocked to see how well I was functioning. My response was that I had never been in war. He told me PTSD is Post Trauma not Post War. I bust out laughing at this and said "decades". I had managed so well within this diagnosis for decades that I didn't realize I had issues.

Post-Traumatic Stress Disorder (PTSD)

There are a lot of reasons, both mental and physical, why a person might be diagnosed with PTSD. It could be as violent as physical abuse, mental abuse, bullying, an animal attack, or a car accident, but it could also be just witnessing someone else's trauma. Anything that your brain considered to be life-threatening is considered traumatic. Triggers for PTSD can happen anywhere: watching TV, standing in your kitchen, attending a party.

Once the damage is done, our brains are constantly on the lookout for signs of trouble in order to protect us. It can be a challenge overcoming PTSD, because you aren't always aware of your unconscious mind's reactions, even when you are in the midst of the physical action itself.

Before learning I had PTSD, I just thought I was your regular corporate mom who did PTA, took kids to soccer, took care of the house, etc... All the stuff that gives you reason to be exhausted the majority of the time. I'd sleep over 8 hours per night yet wake up exhausted, need a pick me up at 4pm and start dozing off at 9:30 pm.

It was explained to me that when you have PTSD your brain is not fully sleeping although your body may be. This is because the brain remains hypervigilant and alert as a self-preservation mechanism. When you sleep properly your body restores itself, your body's organs undergo a kind of cleansing and renewal. Thus, a lack of sleep is detrimental to both your physical and your mental health. So, if you're getting less sleep, you'll eventually experience not just brain fog and cognitive decline. But physical decline as well.

Who Benefit From Using Neurofeedback?

Neurofeedback is not a cure to PTSD, or to any other disorder, but there are still many benefits to be gained. Remember that neurofeedback affects our brains, and as our brains run our entire body, it affects our overall wellbeing, body and mind.

The great thing about neurofeedback is that anyone of any age can benefit from it as there is nothing to succeed or fail at. You just sit and listen to music or watch a video.

I once had a 5 year old girl with selective mutism, who due to anxiety would not speak in public. After 15 sessions this little peanut got up on stage and performed in a play.

Another client, in his 30s, suffered with regular nightmares. After three sessions of neurofeedback, his nightmares started to decrease.

At the end of the day, our brains are the super computers of our body. Regardless of age or gender, when our brains are running optimally, the benefits spill over into so many other areas of our lives.

Neurofeedback Can Bring You Back to Life

We all want to live healthy, happy lives, and so if we are experiencing any kind of disorder, we do whatever we can to manage it. Just like many others, I've tried pharmaceuticals. For the first 18 years of my life, I was on a number of medicines just to keep me alive. Then I realized: yes, medicine was sustaining my life, but it wasn't improving my quality of life. I was surviving, but not thriving. Drugs only treated the symptoms, not the cause. So, I decided to dig down to the heart of what was causing my symptoms, and ultimately, I opted for natural solutions for my physical and a coach for my mental sides.

I think I was so fortunate to have some of the best people on the planet to coach me. Through coaching I understood, logically, what I was supposed to do to feel better, and I would repeat the things that I learned. Yet, I knew that, on a subconscious level, my body was repeating bad habits. Neurofeedback helped me do a better job of establishing healthy mental patterns that brought me back to life.

Where to Get Neurofeedback?

Neurofeedback is available all over the world. I use NeurOptimal, which is the least invasive, and which relies on music—and pauses in music—to interrupt non-optimal patterns allowing your brain to self-correct. And who knows better than your own brain what it needs first and foremost. Other neurofeedback protocol actually has the provider, who does what they think is best for your brain, decide how to train your brain, rather than allowing your brain to decide for itself. Do your own research! Neurofeedback has been in practice since the 1950s, so materials are widely available.

Don't hesitate to try it! Neurofeedback is a great way to have a clearer, balanced mind and a better life.

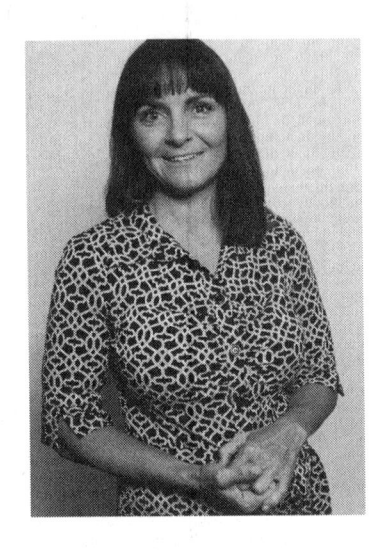

Gina is a Professional and Personal Coach with background experience in training. She coaches individuals and groups towards achieving their goals through ongoing strategy and accountability sessions. She is a graduate of Coach University, the leading global provider of coach training programs as well as a member of the International Coach Federation.

Through no small feat of overcoming serious childhood illness and disability, Gina has become incredibly well versed in wellness and vitality. Given her extensive research and training in the alternative health arena coupled with her Coach University training, Gina brings a broader perspective to whole body health and wellness coaching.

In 2012 she added neurofeedback to her practice as it supports and speeds up work with clients by assisting the brain in breaking out of inefficient patterns; allowing it to run more efficiently, with more resilience, flexibility and stability.

Gina enjoys working with clients on all three levels: physical, psychological, and spiritual. Some clients want all three; some come just for the physical (neurofeedback training).

In her spare time, Gina enjoys assisting her daughters with their Operation NeuroFREEdback Foundation as well as participating in Anthony Robbins events as a Senior Leader.

While Gina's practice is based in Ft. Lauderdale, she does serve South Florida for mobile appointments. For more information, visit www.BrainTrainingForYou.com.

Chapter 6: One Step At A Time

By Stacie Dickerson
Florence, South Carolina

Usually the first question I get when I tell someone what I do is: "What is a life coach?" The answer to that can get a bit complicated, because different life coaches may focus on different things, but essentially a life coach is someone who specializes in working with people to help improve their lives. It could be for business, relationships, fitness, or any other area that a person needs to address in order to improve the quality of their life.

My focus is health and fitness. I've studied this area for many years; it's what I'm most passionate about. I've had the good fortune to attend many different seminars, and I've earned several qualifications and credentials. These include certification through the International Coach Academy, and becoming a strategic intervention coach through the Robbins-Madanes Training Program. I put my training to work helping people all over the U.S. and Canada.

I was drawn to life coaching, and specifically health and fitness life coaching, because of my own personal journey. A number of years ago I found myself putting on a significant amount of weight. I grew up being tall and thin, and I ended up gaining enough weight that I found myself not even recognizing the person looking back at me in the mirror. My self-confidence was extremely low. I spent a lot of my time sitting on the couch, crying and feeling bad about myself. I wasn't happy, but I didn't know why. It was a struggle to come to the realization that my health was a reflection of the anxiety I had in other areas of my life. Finally I decided to take the steps needed to become healthy and fit and that's what I help others do now.

It's All Connected

Coming to the realization that my physical health and fitness were directly connected to how I was feeling emotionally was something that took time. I was "doing" emotions, in a pattern, that weren't helpful. Between my own experiences and the training I've had, it's now my belief that your physical body is really the basis for everything else you do. It's kind of like a springboard for how you act and react in all other areas of your life.

This is even more important when considered with another belief of mine, which is that we're all on this Earth—every one of us—for a reason. Everybody has some mission they were put here to do. We all have unique talents and skills, some combination of things inside of us that make us special. If we squander our abilities by sitting on the couch feeling sick, tired, and depressed, we're never going to be able to live our best lives. Once you start moving— once you see your energy and vitality improve—then you're truly on the path to the greatest personal fulfillment.

One Step at a Time

When I was going through my own struggles I found that things began to change for me when I looked inward. I got tired of feeling the way I did all the time; I wanted something more. I began by asking myself what I wanted to change and how I could affect those changes. I decided that I needed some guidance to move forward, so I found a life coach and eventually got involved with Tony Robbins seminars.

Your journey towards a healthier life begins with small steps. It's really hard to get up one morning and say, "I'm going to be a totally different person today. Everything in my life is now fixed. Here we go!" Maybe that's possible for some people, but most of us aren't able to do that. Sure, you can make an immediate decision to change—but really what you're doing is beginning a shift that will evolve gradually, and maybe imperceptibly, until you look back over your shoulder and see how far you've come.

Take it one thing at a time. Instead of getting overwhelmed with trying a crash diet, just say, "I'm going to start by fixing my breakfasts." Plan your morning meal, set a goal to be at a certain calorie count and nutritional level, and once you've done that, celebrate the victory. From there you can continue to challenge yourself by improving your lunch, then your snacks, your dinner, and your water intake. Eventually you're at the point where you're in the habit of doing all of these things, but it doesn't happen overnight. Take the first step, be happy with your successes along the way, and continue to challenge yourself.

Simple Isn't the Same as Easy

The "one step at a time" method sounds pretty simple, and that's because it is. We tend to overcomplicate things. Most things that work tend to come from very simple ideas—but being simple just describes an idea that's easy to understand, and not necessarily one that's easy to implement. It's not easy to recognize that there's a problem in your life. Sometimes it's not easy to find the determination to take those first steps and maybe make some sacrifices along the way. It's not easy saying you need help getting where you want to go, and it's not easy figuring out where you want to go in the first place.

One thing that can make the process a little easier in the long run is making sure that you're taking the time to set achievable goals. We call them S.M.A.R.T. goals: Specific, Measurable, Action-oriented, Reasonable, and Timed.

When you set a goal, you want it to be as <u>specific</u> and detailed as possible so you can really visualize it. You want to be able to <u>measure</u> your progress in achieving that goal, which is like celebrating those small steps and milestones. You want your goals to be <u>action-oriented</u> so that you can take action yourself in order to achieve them. Your goal has to be <u>reasonable</u>, like changing one meal at a time instead of overhauling your entire kitchen. Finally, "<u>timed</u>" means that you want to have an idea of how long it will take you to reach your goals, a deadline.

The process of setting S.M.A.R.T. goals will help set you up for success regardless of what those goals are. It will give you time to really think about which goals are important to you and why. It will also let you think about what will be different in your life as a result of working toward and achieving those goals. How will your home life be better if you're able to be more active with your family? If you take care of your health and fitness so you can be around longer to spend more time with your family, how will that affect them? What happens if you don't take action? These types of goals let you get fully invested in your decision because you understand why you're doing what you're doing. You don't want goals to push you. You want your goals to be pulling you towards them, drawing you towards your future.

Know Why to Know How

There are so many different diet and fitness plans out there these days, and thanks to the Internet it's never been easier to research them. There's the whole foods plant-based diet, the Mediterranean diet, the Paleo diet, and many more. There's even a grapefruit diet. People always seem to wonder which program is right for them because they hear about a friend who has great success with something and then another friend who didn't get anywhere with the exact same plan. The bottom line is that in order to find out how you can achieve success in any plan you have to understand why you're starting a plan in the first place. Reasons come first; how second.

I've expressed that setting goals is an important part of finding your best life possible, and that relates here as well. Health and fitness are all about strategies; those are the "how." However, I can't help develop strategies for you if you don't know why you're looking for them.

If I ask you why you've come to see me and you say you want to be healthier, that leaves a lot of wiggle room. Do you mean you want to lose weight? Do you mean you want to gain muscle? Do you want to lower your blood pressure? Even the common reason of, "I just want to eat healthier" isn't enough of a "why." Are you feeling tired, so you want more energy? Are you an endurance athlete who needs a high performance diet? Are you looking to change your diet because you want to be cruelty-free or vegan? "Healthy" means different things in different contexts, so taking the time to really understand why you're making a change will help tremendously in strategizing how to make those changes as beneficial as possible.

Living Healthy

I'm living, breathing proof of how beneficial it can be to be truly healthy, and how getting your health in line affects every aspect of your life. You become healthy on the inside and out, mentally and physically, and you're able to feel more fulfilled every day because you can do more, give more. If you're ready to take the first steps toward your own best life, start by being very clear about what "best life" and "truly healthy" mean to you. Ultimately, it comes down to being happy, so first decide what mental, physical, and spiritual health and happiness look like in your own mind. Remember: if you don't know what your goals are, you won't know when you reach them.

My final piece of advice is to get a coach. Find someone that will hold your feet to the fire and hold you accountable for the things you say you'll do, but who will also hold your hand as you go through the process. Good coaches are non-judgmental and will talk straight with you. They're not your friend, so they won't sugar coat things or tell you what you want to hear. They'll be your coach and will work hard to see you reach the goals that are important to you. I can tell you that having a coach has made a tremendous impact in my own life and I can't recommend it enough for others.

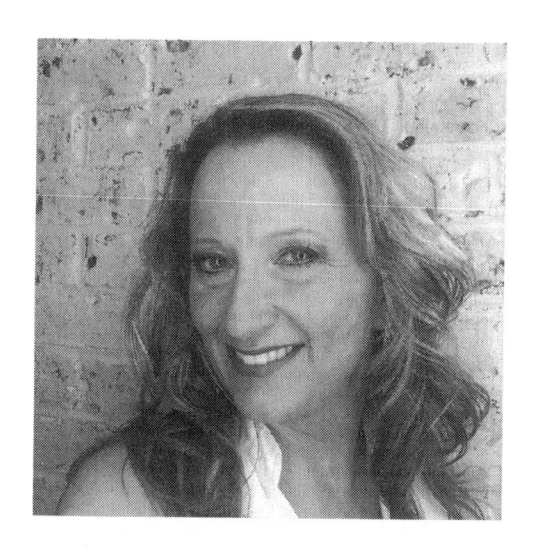

Stacie Dickerson is an Anthony Robbins Results coach, a certified Strategic Intervention Life Coach through Robbins-Madanes Training Center, and a Certified Life Coach through the International Coach Academy. She is a contributing author in the anthology SMART Women Embrace Transitions: How to Lean Into Change with Your Body Mind and Soul.

As a coach she specializes in the areas of business and health & fitness.

She has over 20 years of experience in the management and marketing of shopping centers and holds numerous certifications through the International Council of Shopping Centers, including CRX, CSM and CMD. In addition to being a former gym owner, she has a background as a personal trainer through the National Academy of Sports Medicine, and as a nutritional counselor through APEX Nutrition.

She is the founder of The Healthy Lifestyle Institute, an organization committed to helping people with the mental side of living a healthy lifestyle so they can live with energy, confidence and purpose.

Connect with Stacie at www.HealthyLifestyleInstitute.co, www.ExcuseBusters.club or on Facebook at www.facebook.com/HealthyLifestyleInstitute

Chapter 7: Mindfulness & Meditation

By Shaleena Anand
London, United Kingdom

I think most Millennials can relate to my story because our lives progressed along a similar trajectory—normal family upbringing, university, friends. My degree was in Linguistics & Communications. I enjoyed the student years, like most of us, although I had no clear concept of what I wanted from life after I graduated. After University I felt stuck in the rut of a job I didn't really like; I was stressed out and suffering bouts of anxiety. Like a lot of us, I kept asking myself, "Is this all there is to life?" That is the point from which I started my spiritual journey: rock bottom. I climbed back up from there. I tried many forms of meditation, but when I found I preferred Deepak Chopra's teachings, I decided to get accredited by the Chopra Center.

But my journey really sped up when I decided to create on my own.

Why the Emphasis on Millennials?

Mindfulness meditations lie on a spiritual path that has existed for thousands of years. They are important and relevant to people of any age; these teachings and practices are in use all around the world.

But I have a soft spot for Millennials. I remember how tough it was growing up even in the best of times—the difficulties with my mental health state, and the lack of help designed for people of my age and upbringing, help that was relevant and made sense to me. I saw that Millennials were an untouched area, disconnected from spirituality so I felt I could help lots of people. Our culture often ignores the fact that young people are stressed out and, therefore, little is done to help us battle stress and anxiety.

We think about stress in terms of corporate ladders and backstabbing, kids and mortgages to worry about. We associate stress and anxiety with later years in life. It is true that people well into their careers tend to be swamped by problems to such an extent that they can no longer relate to the complexities and worries of the younger generations. However, personal relations, schools and exams put a lot of pressure on the youth, creating a lot of stress. I believe that growing up is the perfect time to nip that stress in the bud by teaching young people mindfulness and meditation—making spirituality a part of their personality, a part of their daily regimen.

I used to think my life was very 'normal'. In college, I surrounded myself with other people who also had a negative perception of life as I used too. Our conversations usually revolved around who had the worst day and expressing our strong feelings of unfulfillment for the lives we were living.

Our generation has gotten caught up in not looking at our glass being half-full, or even overflowing. We don't want to come across as egotistical. That practice of self-censoring any positive remarks about ourselves fascinated me. Where did all that self-abnegation come from?

The Difference Between Millennials and Older Generations

The first and most obvious difference between Millennials and, say, Baby Boomers, is the technological advances—the tablets and smart phones that we all have now. Social media wields incredible power over us. Research shows that social media, as amazing a phenomenon that it is, is the root of a lot of anxiety and stress for young people. Social media helps us connect with people, but it also helps create a disconnect for many of us. It is very unhealthy to feel that your self-worth depends on how many likes or followers you get. If you post an article on Facebook about something interesting to you but no one "likes" it, it's easy to feel like you were wrong, that you shouldn't have been interested to begin with. That is nonsense, of course.

My Story

I grew up in a Hindu household, and I have been aware of the practice of meditation since I was very young. Of course, as I was also growing up in face paced Western society, it all kind of fizzled out; but, as I now understand, the practice stayed with me unconsciously. So I can say that I've been meditating most of my life—in the past mostly unknowingly, but a lot more consciously recently.

When I was young I viewed myself as healthy, because I was slim. I didn't look unhealthy. It seems that society keeps telling us that the only way you can be unhealthy is when you are overweight. That is not true. I was not overweight and looked fine except for the acne that I chose to ignore, but I did not feel fine. Something inside of me just felt incomplete. Looking back at that period now, I see that acne was the way my body was screaming out for help. I didn't know then but now I know that skin is the first place toxins are released from. So, although I was not putting on weight, all those toxins were coming out through my skin.

The turning point has come to me after years of build-up, when all my mental and physical toxicity started integrating itself into my personality. I truly believed that I was angry, depressed, or anxious purely because that was my personality and those were my unique personality traits. All my friends were in a similar condition. We were all unwittingly strengthening each other's belief that we simply were that way by nature. I did not really think anything was wrong with me until I read a book by Deepak Chopra called The Seven Spiritual Laws of Success. After I read it, I realized that there was a different way to live my life.

Only now that a meditation regimen is a part of my life and I teach it to others, do I understood how vital it is to take the time every day to quiet yourself and listen to what your body and your mind are telling you.

Before I simply thought that by nature I wasn't very lovable; I was often angry and impatient with people, but that was just me, my personality. Now I know better. Now, I never raise my voice at anyone. I don't get angry. I feel completely fine. All I did to achieve that was going back to basics, asking myself questions like: "Why am I here?" "What is my purpose?" "How can I help others?"

Now I know that my mission in life is to help other people. I think the main thing that you have to understand—and mindfulness and meditations really will help—is that you do not need to fix yourself. Nobody is broken, so we do not need to be fixed. In order to help yourself, you simply need to get to know yourself better. The only way to do that is to listen to the little voice in your head and become attuned to what the energy you are immersed in is saying to you.

Meditations

Meditation is not just sitting quietly. It's a spiritual process that can be uniquely tailor-made to suit different people. I am a believer in changing the practice to suit the client. I am not sure everyone would agree with me on that, but it is my personal belief. With younger people in particular, it makes more sense to do what they feel more comfortable with. So I practice a range of different meditations. I do a silent meditation when you work on your breathing, count your breathing, simply try clear your thoughts. I use Pranayama breathing techniques to do that.

Breathe in through your nose and your mouth. Fill up your stomach like a hot air balloon. Then hold. Count 1, 2, 3, 4, 5. Then breathe out. Let your diaphragm expel all that air. Breathe in again; count 1, 2, 3, 4, 5, and release. Just focus on that breathing. This is great for beginners.

The main thing to remember that there is no right or wrong way to meditate. The entire purpose of meditation is to bring you back to basics.

One practice we offer is guided meditation, where I run a class and speak to my students through a meditation. I encourage them to think about what their purpose in life is and why they are here.

I also practice primordial sound meditation, a technique created by the Chopra Center.

I always urge my students to not prejudge a meditation, and discourage them from starting a meditation expecting miraculous results (like levitation). The attitude I teach is just do it, just meditate, remembering that you are doing it for yourself.

I also tell my students to not focus on not thinking about anything—because the more you try not to think about something, the more you're going to think about it! I guide them to concentrate their attention on their breathing. Just concentrate on your breathing, slowly, slowly. If a thought comes to mind, that is fine; let the thought come and go. Don't judge it. Don't try to decide whether it's positive or negative. Any emotions attached to your thoughts will also come and go.

Special postures aren't necessary, either. What is important is to assume a body position that is comfortable. If you don't feel comfortable sitting cross-legged on the floor, then sit on a chair. If you want to lie down, do it—just not on your bed. You do not want to string that mental connection between meditating and sleeping. Otherwise, anything goes. No need to sit cross-legged just so, or go to a temple. The important thing is to simply start meditating and do it in a comfortable position.

I recommend 20-minute meditations to beginners. Many teachers insist on 30-minute sessions, but I believe that changes can be made to suit the client and 20-minute meditation works best when working with young clients. Twenty minutes is not too long to be difficult, but you still get enough benefits from that amount of time. If after ten minutes you are up and away, thinking it isn't for you and it wasn't working anyway and you didn't like it, try again in a few hours, and again, until you get a positive result. You don't want meditations becoming an unwelcome chore for you. You want to look forward to your meditation sessions.

Meditating twice a day produces best results. Do it first thing in the morning. Wake up, empty your bladder, brush your teeth, then go sit down wherever it is you usually meditate and do your 20 minutes or 10 minutes or for however long you've allocated the time.

Meditate again a couple of hours before you go to sleep—maybe even before your evening meal. Avoid meditating on a full stomach—but don't meditate on an empty stomach! If you meditate hungry, your entire session will be dedicated to the feeling of hunger; your body will divert all your energy to the stomach. Similarly, if you meditate on a full stomach, the opposite will happen and you will end up quietly asleep or lethargic.

Returning to guided meditations: with very large groups, I like to keep it simple. I have three questions that I keep repeating, getting them to work through the content. My goal is to bring participants back to what I think of as the "human basics," such as knowing why we are here as a human race, what we are supposed to do, and how they can help. I've seen how these questions can be life-changing.

The first question is, "Just ask yourselves, 'Who am I?'" I am always amazed by what comes to people's heads when they are put on the spot this way.

The next question I ask them is, "What do I want? What do I want from life?"

The third one is, "What is my purpose? What is my Dharma?" Dharma is kind of like "duty." What is my dharma for being here?"

I try to keep these guided sessions to 20-30 minutes. I have done hour-long meditations as well, but they would only be suitable for those who had done meditations before.

A few words about the primordial sound meditations, founded by Deepak Chopra and the Chopra Center. In this form of meditation you do not let out any sound out loud; you create an internal sound that the universe was making at the exact time and place of your birth. It's an internal chanting meditation. The exact sound is calculated by the Chopra Center. When they work out the sound, they give it to you and you use it in meditations from that point on. That sound is a secret; it's yours alone. You don't share it with anybody. You never say it aloud. It is a personal connection between your mind, body, and soul. The only time this sound is made out loud is when your instructor is giving it to you. It is a very special moment that you share with your instructor, because you feel a kind of a special recognition when you hear your mantra; you have a feeling that you heard that exact sound before. Obviously, that is the Universe speaking.

To you that sound means, "I am." It gives you a sense of going back to your starting point and realizing that we are all from the Universe. We use "I am" a lot in meditations. It really means, "I am the Universe" or "I am a part of the Universe." You begin seeing that we are all just one pool of energy that is recycled again and again and that really we are all one living, breathing thing. It is really amazing.

Who Needs to Meditate?

All people benefit immensely from regular meditation, but some of us do need it more than others. For example, if you are having trouble concentrating you should start meditating. You would probably need to meditate more than others, just because at the beginning the practice often feels uncomfortable. That sense of discomfort is your mind and your body releasing the toxins inside of you. I have a lot of clients who come to me and say that they didn't have a very good session, they didn't like it, it wasn't working for them. And I always tell them to keep going, push through it, carry on, try it again, do it like a challenge. And if they push through it, they always enjoy it.

Benefits of Meditation

When people hear the word "meditation" they usually think about relaxation and stress reduction, and they are right—meditations do help with that 100%.   But I really believe it is important to understand that meditations help with actual physical illnesses as well.

I had a client who suffered from rheumatoid arthritis, which is a disease considered incurable by medical science. The body is attacking itself, so to speak. She was prescribed Methotrexate to prevent swelling of the joints. Her neck and her knees would swell up quite a lot, which is a part of that illness.

She meditated under my supervision once a week for three months. Then I sent her home for 21 days to meditate daily on her own. And after that she hasn't had to take her pills even once. Six months have passed, no pills. I think it is amazing.

There are many examples of, and even studies about, different ways that meditations help people with terminal illnesses. In many cases you cannot stop a terminal illness, but you can definitely prolong life.

Some people seem to have a problem with finding time to meditate. They say that meditating in a group is good because they arrive specifically to meditate using the time dedicated to meditation, but finding time to meditate on their own is a near impossibility. In my eyes, this problem is an artificial challenge, created specifically as an excuse not to meditate. So I think you need to work out your "Why" for meditating and make it absolutely clear to yourself. You must be dead certain why you are doing it. I would not leave my house without brushing my teeth, just the same way as I wouldn't leave my house without meditating. You have to make sure it is that strong of a feeling in you.

We often say we want something, like an improved health or a better mental parity, but we do not get obsessed with how to attain it. With meditation, you almost have to become obsessed in order to do it. The challenge is to get my clients to realize how useful it is and how much they can get out of it. With meditations and mindfulness, the proof is in the pudding. So when people experience and understand things, see the results, do it under your supervision and then on their own, from that point on it's smooth sailing.

The First Step

The first step for a person is to say, "Yes, I want to start meditating." And then try it on your own. The web is an amazing tool, full of practical how-to articles and demonstrations. If you find it interesting and useful, then find a professional, an expert in the field, and go learn more from them.

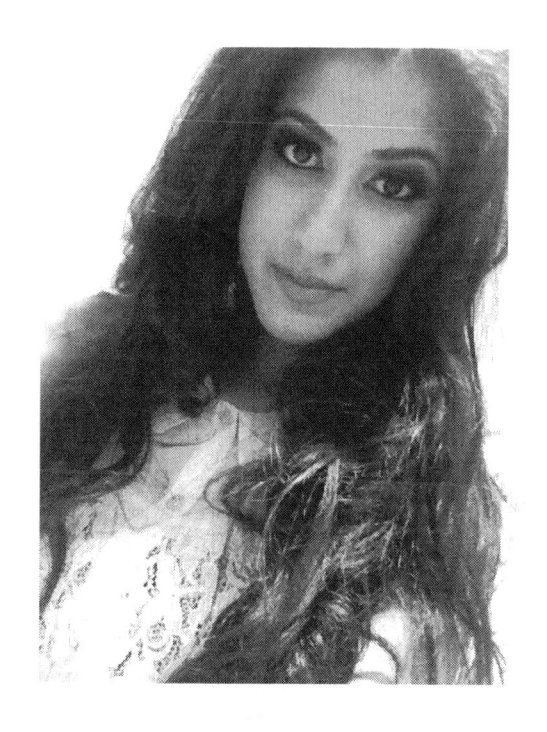

Shaleena Anand is a meditation & mindfulness consultant. She has extensively studied communications and neuro-linguistic programming which she incorporates into her sessions. Shaleena is the founder of WIIDLO: 'What if I don't like oysters?'- an online platform for people to overcome the 'what if' moments in their lives.

For more information, visit www.wiidlo.com.

Chapter 8:
The Eat Bacon Diet

By Mark Niemchak, D.C.
Raleigh, North Carolina

Hello. I'm Dr. Mark Niemchak, chiropractor, functioning nutritionist and promoter of lifestyle advocacy. I have been a chiropractor for 33 years. I've also had experience as a paramedic, an EMT, a physician's assistant, and years of experience working with medical doctors, psychologist, physical therapist, massage therapist, and other people in the health and wellness industry. I feel that my pursuit of the ultimate truth in lifestyle and wellness practices is of incredible value to people to obtain optimal health. This is best accomplished by controlling what you eat. I therefore recommend a ketogenic diet.

So, what actually is a ketogenic diet? Some people may think that a ketogenic diet is a fad diet and the most notable ketogenic diet experience was Dr. Adkins, when in actuality, a ketogenic diet was the diet every person on this planet followed prior to agriculture being introduced. A ketogenic diet is primarily a diet where, instead of your body using glucose to fuel your body, you use the fat in your body as a fuel source. When you eat in a ketogenic fashion, you eat high-fat, moderate protein, and extremely low carbohydrates. Below, you will find details of a ketogenic diet, and how to best implement it in your life.

The Eat Bacon Diet

This diet focuses on providing your body with the nutrition it needs, such as protein and fats, while limiting the foods that you don't need, in the form of carbohydrates. This would be all carbohydrates including vegetable and fruits. For this diet to be most effective, you will need to keep your total carbohydrates to *less than 20 grams per day*. This is why it is extremely important to track everything you put in your mouth good or bad.

Here's another concept key to the success of this diet:
When you are hungry, eat. When you are not hungry, do not *eat.*

Foods that you can eat:

Meat: hamburger, steaks, pork, bacon, sausage, ham, veal, lamb, pepperoni, hot dogs, lunch meats or other meats, etc. (Make sure to take into consideration that carbohydrates are in some items like sausage, hot dogs and ham, just make sure to keep track of them.)

Poultry: Chicken, turkey, duck or other fowl.

Fish & Shellfish: Any fish including tuna, salmon, catfish, bass, trout, shrimp, scallops, crabs and lobster. (Nothing with breading on it)

Eggs: Whole eggs are not restricted at all, but it is important to eat the whole egg as the yoke has the fat and nutrition that you need most.

Key: *Don't avoid the fat!* Cook with real butter, olive oil, coconut oil, avocado oil or animal fat oils, like your bacon fat drippings.

What about salad?

Yes on this diet *you can* eat a salad every day. However you should limit the greens to *no more than 2 cups per day.*

Salad items include: arugula, bok choy, cabbage, chard, chives, endive, greens (i.e. beets, collards, mustard and turnips) kale, all types of lettuce, parsley, spinach, radicchio, Radishes, scallions and watercress, *IF IT IS A LEAF, YOU CAN IT IN MODERATION.*

What about other vegetables?

You can *eat up to 1 cup* (measured uncooked) no starch vegetables a day.

Vegetables included: artichokes, asparagus, broccoli, Brussels sprouts, cauliflower, celery, cucumber, eggplant, green beans, jicama, leeks, mushrooms, okra, onions, peppers, tomatoes, shallots, snow peas, sprouts, sugar snap peas, summer squash, rhubarb, wax beans and zucchini.

Just remember, all vegetables contain carbohydrates, so track carefully.

What about fruit?

It is best to avoid all fruits as the carbohydrates are high and increase your carb cravings.

Foods that are allowed in limited quantities:

Cheese: *do not eat more than 4 ounces a day.* These cheeses include Swiss, cheddar, brie, camembert, blue, mozzarella, Gruyere, cream cheese, goat cheese and parmesan cheese. *No fat-free or low-fat cheeses, as these are loaded with sugar.*

Cream: no more than 2 tablespoons per day. This includes heavy, light or sour cream. This does not include half and half or milk. Whipping cream is acceptable as long as no sugar has been added.

Mayonnaise: no more than 2 tablespoons per day.
Olives: no more than 6 a day (black or green)
Avocado: no more than ½ an avocado a day.
Soy sauces: no more than 2 tablespoons a day
Pickles: no more than 2 servings a day. (dill or sugar-free) always read the label first.

Zero and low carb snacks: sugar-free jello, pork rinds, deviled eggs, pepperoni slices and lunch meats.

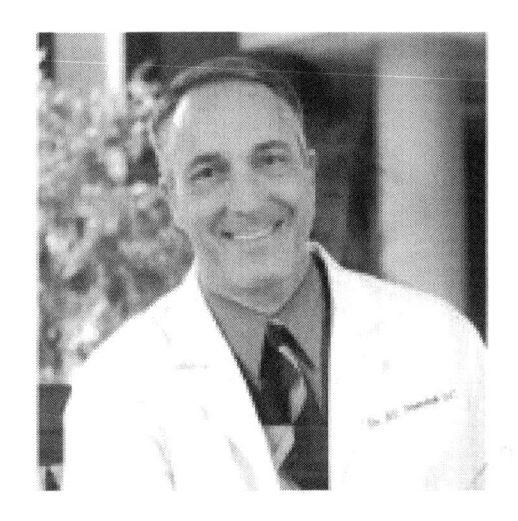

Mark Niemchak is a Doctor of Chiropractic based in Raleigh, North Carolina.

Once overweight and unhealthy, Niemchak started looking more closely at his nutrition, his movement, and his mindset. He made shifts in his life, embracing Lifestyle Medicine. His own physical transformation is an example of the work he does with his patients.

For more information, visit www.ideallifestyleadvocates.com.

Chapter 9: Fitness Failed Me

By Ross Johnson
Boulder, Colorado

There's a problem with the world of fitness. A problem plaguing students, teachers, trainers, practitioners, and everyone in between.

What is the problem?

Everything.

Modern fitness is the *definition* of chaos. Look at all the people and programs dispensing advice—the books, podcasts, DVDs, YouTube videos, magazines, and blogs. It's mind-numbing and confusing. All these sources, these experts, they're all saying different things. They're all contradicting each other. It's inefficient. It's overwhelming.

And it makes true learning, true physical development, *impossible*. How do I know? Because I spent years living in the very heart of the chaos.

Once upon a time, I was completely absorbed by the myths of modern fitness culture. In fact, I was so enveloped—so far down the rabbit hole—that I cut a massive check to a college in the hopes of becoming a certified personal trainer.

I was convinced that earning this little paper certificate would allow me to understand *everything* there was to know about health and fitness. It would enable me to become a *master* of my body and, in doing so, gain the knowledge, wisdom, and technique to help people become masters of theirs.

Unfortunately, the lessons I'd discover while in school were very much to the contrary. In fact, there were no lessons, just contradictions. Books saying my instructors were wrong. Instructors saying my books were wrong. It was nothing short of an educational nightmare.

Having said all that, I'm extremely glad I paid all that money for school because, had I not, I never would have learned the most important lesson of all:

When it comes to being healthy, there is no ONE path--no RIGHT path-- there is only YOUR path. Find it and stick to it.

Ninety-five percent of the people in the world of "certified" fitness run on a single-speed mental treadmill. They operate on that *"It's my way or the highway"* mentality. But that's the exact *opposite* of what fitness teachers and coaches should be doing. They should be encouraging students like you to try different approaches, try new things. Do whatever it takes to discover a pathway to fitness that works for you. And when you find that pathway, it's your instructor's responsibility to help you zero in on it. To give it all their effort and energy, or, if need be, to help you find a new instructor who can offer true expertise in your chosen field.

I'm fortunate to have found a method and a mentor that work for me. And since I started committing to that one technique and a single coach, my progress has skyrocketed.

But it wasn't always this way.

Meet the Meathead

I have a confession to make. Once upon a time, I was a meathead.

Not even a casual, part-time meathead. I'm talking a full-time, full-on "bro." To work out, I'd max out my bench, go for broke on sit-ups, and pound my knees on the treadmill for 20 minutes a day to make sure I was getting the cardio necessary for a "whole-body" workout.

I wanted the six-pack abs. I wanted the bulging arms. I was convinced this practice of punitively pumping iron was the single path to perfection, both on the inside and out.

Why? Because that was the culture of my age group, and it was the culture encouraged by the professionals at my gym. It's pretty humbling to revisit those days in my head, because my whole attitude to fitness has changed so dramatically.

I was following the crowd without a care in the word.

And—honestly?—I was OK with following the crowd, because I loved the idea of working out, I loved heading to the gym every day not necessarily to lift, but to grind. I knew in my heart that my life was going to revolve around exercise, I knew health and fitness were my calling.

But I also knew that if I was going to make a life out of health and fitness, I needed to learn more—a lot more—than what was being taught at my weightlifting-centric gym.

So when all of my friends left our middle-of-nowhere hometown for college, I decided to focus all of my energy on becoming a fitness know-it-all, and what better way to do that then become a certified personal trainer?

An application, an interview, and a massive deposit check later, I was enrolled at a well-known health and wellness school, ready to become Ross Johnson – Certified Personal Trainer and fitness aficionado.

A world-shattering wake-up

For the next six months, I was a full-time student with a brutal 6-day schedule:
- Wake up at 5:30AM
- Drive 2+ hours to school
- Attend class for 5 hours
- Drive 2+ hours home
- Go straight to work as a pizza delivery guy until 9:00pm
- Go home and go to sleep

But becoming a certified personal trainer was going to give me all the insight I'd need—not only to discover my path, but to become a practitioner of health and wellness wisdom for the world—so I was willing to make the sacrifice. Each day I walked into the classroom dog-tired but undaunted, ready to soak up anything my instructors had to offer.

In fact, my passion for health and wellness—about a future of making a difference in people's lives—reached such a fever pitch following my enrollment that I started going beyond our core curriculum. I was reading anything, and I do mean *anything*, I could get my hands on. I bought books, magazines, and journals on every fitness-related subject you could possibly imagine, and read, and read, and read. You know how people binge watch a TV series on Netflix? Yeah, that's what I was doing with all this health and fitness literature.

This supplemental education should have been a real complement to everything I was learning in school but, unfortunately, it was quite the opposite. I went from walking out of class every day thinking "That's amazing," to walking out of class every day thinking, "That's bullshit." The information I was consuming like an absolute addict would, more often than not, directly conflict with what I was learning in the classroom.

Keep in mind, the information that I was extracting from these extracurricular books wasn't written by crackpots or random hacks with a WordPress blog; these were published authors with real credentials. I'm talking M.D.s, Ph.D.s, PTs, CPTs.

When I'd raise an objection, or challenge my teachers on any of this conflicting information, they would first validate my point and completely confirm the accuracy of what I was learning outside of class.

But after that validation, they would inform me that I shouldn't waste my time learning outside the classroom because only the answers covered in class would be considered "right" when it came time for the NASM Certification Test—the test needed to gain my personal trainer certification. It was mind-boggling to be told, "Both A and B are correct, but when it comes time for the test, only A will be correct, so it's best to forget about B."

How could two totally different answers be simultaneously be right? Even more confusing, how could only one of the "right" answers actually be "right" on the test?

I went into this educational adventure expecting complete, unquestionable health and fitness knowledge, but by the time graduation rolled around, the only thing I knew with certainty was this: the fitness industry—from education to execution—was very, very confused.

Finding my path

Ask a CrossFit coach about the best way to learn a handstand. Then ask a yoga instructor. Then a gymnast, followed by a martial artist, followed by a personal trainer. I can 100% guarantee you'll get a different but "definitive" answer every time.

Each expert is confident their technique is not only the best option, but the only option. They're all experts, they can all do a handstand, but they're all saying different things. Just like my teachers in school, just like the authors of the books I was reading, and just like the National Academy of Sports Medicine who made the certification test I needed to pass.

How can they all of these experts be right and wrong at the same time? This is at the very heart of what's plaguing the fitness industry: conflict. Ask three different Certified Personal Trainers about the best way to get a six-pack, and you're going to get three different answers.

So what's the solution? Well, there's no simple one.

You need to start by outlining your goals—*what do you want?* Washboard abs? The ability to execute a handstand? The strength to squat 500 pounds?

Hold that want, that goal, in your mind, because that's going to become the center of your universe. Then start trying things—classes, coaches, workouts, gyms—paying attention to what you like versus what you don't. Do not let yourself get pressured by the latest craze or fad; just pay attention to what you feel. When you find a coach, class, or program that really resonates, hold onto it.

My breakthrough came from Ido Portal.

Ido's an Israeli movement teacher whose journey was quite reflective of mine. He began with a passion for fitness and little else. That passion led him on a quest for education—for universal health and fitness truth. What he learned instead was that the entire fitness industry is broken. Eventually, Ido decided his only recourse for achieving true health and fitness was through movement—and that realization motivated him to construct his own method for physical human development.

Everything Ido taught resonated with me. In the mad information maze of health and fitness advice, I'd found a mentor and method I could really latch on to.

This was my turning point. This was when I discovered the true secret to health and fitness wasn't rooted in any certification, book, or specific technique, it was rooted in finding something that spoke to you as a human. I joined a class and began practicing Ido's method, and in two months I had improved more in my own physical development than I had in years of practicing other techniques.

Find a Technique, Find a Teacher

I'm not sharing this story because I want you to start practicing the Ido Portal Method; I'm sharing it to show the importance of finding a single method and teacher that resonates with you. Devoting yourself to a single teacher or coach makes a huge difference in how effectively you learn. It changes how your brain responds to the environment, making you more aware, more receptive, and more capable of forming the permanent neural connections that solidify new skills.

I took a big risk to immerse myself in Ido's teaching: I packed up my life and moved across the country to train with one of his disciples, Matt Bernstein.

Even though I had never met Matt, I joined his class in the hopes of soaking up all the knowledge I possibly could—he was going to be the conduit through which I could further accomplish my goals. My mission was to get better at Ido's method, and using Matt as my single source of education and input was going to be the most effective and efficient means of getting where I wanted to be.

Now, you don't need to move across the country to become a master of your body, but if you're serious about your health and fitness goals, you need to subscribe to one method and one teacher. Find your method, then find your coach—listen to what is said, then do the work and do it mercilessly.

Direct your energy. Hone your focus. And you'll secure the results you want much faster.

When it all pays off...

Earlier, I specifically referenced a handstand.

The handstand is one of those skills I'd always wanted to master, but <u>never</u> had been able to in all my days of working out. I'd walk past guys and gals in the park on a sunny afternoon doing straight-as-a-plank handstands in the grass, and find myself supremely jealous.

I tried for months and months to perform an applause-worthy handstand, but never could because I was constantly taking advice from different coaches, trainers, and experts. I trawled YouTube for videos, joined Facebook groups, followed CrossFit bloggers, read dozens of how-to's on Reddit. But no matter how much I "learned" handstands, I couldn't improve—my handstand was less of a straight, sturdy plank, and more of wobbly, "I'm-about-to-fall-on-my-face" human question mark.

I struggled, not because I lacked the discipline, commitment, or natural skill, but because there was too much conflicting instruction coming in for me to ever get close to consistency in execution. I was so eager to learn that I was just consuming too much information.

What one person advised, another person would warn against. When one article promised would help me in a matter of weeks, another article told me would damage my wrists and posture. I'd try one method for a week or two, and when it didn't work, I'd give up and move on to something else. My inability to commit a program, and therefore a coach, inhibited me from making the progress I so desperately wanted.

Yet, when I confined myself to a single source of instruction? A method of training that <u>really</u> spoke to me as an individual? Yep, you guessed it: I nailed it.

A kick-ass handstand was one of the very first things I learned to not only do, but do well, after about four weeks of training exclusively with Matt. I was focusing on a single technique, a single coach, and a single voice. My foundations—wrist strength and spine position—developed rapidly under Matt's tutelage, and within two-months I was not only able to do a straight-line handstand, but hold it for 60 seconds.

It's a lesson you can apply to any fitness goal, whether it's handstands, back squats, or weight loss. It takes formulaic practice and coaching to build the strength and neural connections necessary to become truly skilled.

Constantly chopping and changing your technique means retarding your overall progress—the mind and body don't know what they're supposed to be remembering, which means the learning process never truly starts. Repetition and focus are the best ways to master a new discipline, which is why I say to find your goal, find your path, find your coach, and then stick to them.

The Science Behind It All

When people start talking skill development and mastery, there's a number that gets thrown around a lot: 10,000 hours.

There's this perception—in my opinion, totally misguided—that mastery requires a heavy investment of time.

The problem is that time is far and away the average person's most valuable resource—it is decidedly finite, we are given a fixed amount, and it is impossible to generate more.

But I've come to the conclusion that mastering a skill is not really about the minutes or hours spent; it's about the performance of the right repetitions.

Think back to your time in elementary school. Your teacher undoubtedly made you perform countless repetitions of your basic 12 by 12 times table. These repetitions were performed rigorously and for a period of time, but that period of time was less than 10,000 hours—in fact, it was probably less than 100. Yet, now, when someone pulls you aside and says, "hey, what's two times three?" you immediately and unconsciously reply "six."

There's a reason why the repetition builds speed and skill so effectively: when you repeat an action over and over, you actually change the structure of your brain. Whether it's reciting your times table or executing a biceps curl with perfect form, you're delivering the same instructions across the same neural pathways. As those signals are repeated, thicker myelin—a vital neurological substance comprised of essential fatty acids—starts to build up between the nerve cells in the brain. Myelin acts as the highway between nerve cells: the thicker the myelin, the faster your brain signals can travel across your neural pathways.

With everyday repetition, these pathways get clearer, wider, and easier to travel along. That's why two times three is such an easy operation: because you've done it so many times, the myelin in your brain is thick. The "pathway" is clear and you can perform the operation without any conscious thought.

Repetition builds skill with anything. At first, my attempts at a perfect handstand seemed impossible. I'd put my hands down, pick my feet up off the ground, and invert, before quickly losing balance and toppling over. But even the most complicated movements can be broken down into a series of simple, easily replicable progressions. The more you execute these foundational movements, the better you condition your neuromuscular structure, and the better you become.

But repetition isn't without its risks—it only leads to success if you're repeating the right messages, instructions, and actions. If you do something incorrectly, your brain and body will remember incorrect patterns. The myelin in your brain can't distinguish between a pathway that's helping you and one that's holding you back—what you repeat is what you get.

That's why it's so important to establish your goal, find a method of practice that speaks to who you are, and then find a single instructor to help you along the way. Find the teacher who'll train you in techniques that are right for you. Do that, and you'll start building the pathways that lead to success. Don't do it, and you'll only build pathways that you'll have to destroy (unlearn) down the road. Start leveraging the power of repetition to train your brain and body and you'll find that you can learn absolutely anything.

Where to Go From Here?

At this point, you know my story. You know why finding the right path, your path, to health and wellness is important. You understand the value of repetition. And you can see why finding a teacher, instructor, or coach that you can truly buy into is critical. But I haven't yet told you how to find that teacher.

Look for somebody who's "been there, done that." An individual who has not only accomplished that which you are seeking to accomplish, but done so within the framework of your preferred methodology.

My goal was to become a master of fitness, and the method of fitness that most readily spoke to me was the Ido Portal method, so I went and found a coach (Matt Bernstein) who could show me the way. I never asked Matt directly to be my mentor—we never even discussed the topic of mentorship—but it happened because I knew he was the conduit to achieving my fitness-related goals.

When I met him for the first time, I told Matt I moved to Boulder, Colorado with the sole purpose of training with him. I told him point-blank that I wanted what he currently had: to be a supremely talented student of the Ido Portal Method. I went out of my way to show Matt that I was doing the work and taking his lessons seriously. That dedication and loyalty to his instruction has helped us form a fantastic bond, and that bond has only amplified my ability to learn.

When you're looking for the right mentor or coach, remember that all teachers want committed students, and all students want committed teachers. If you can focus on a goal, express a willingness to do the work, and unequivocally commit yourself to learning process, you will find a mentor. Focus on learning from them; help them; and be the student that they've been looking for. Identify your objective, find your path, pinpoint your teacher, and you will hit your goal.

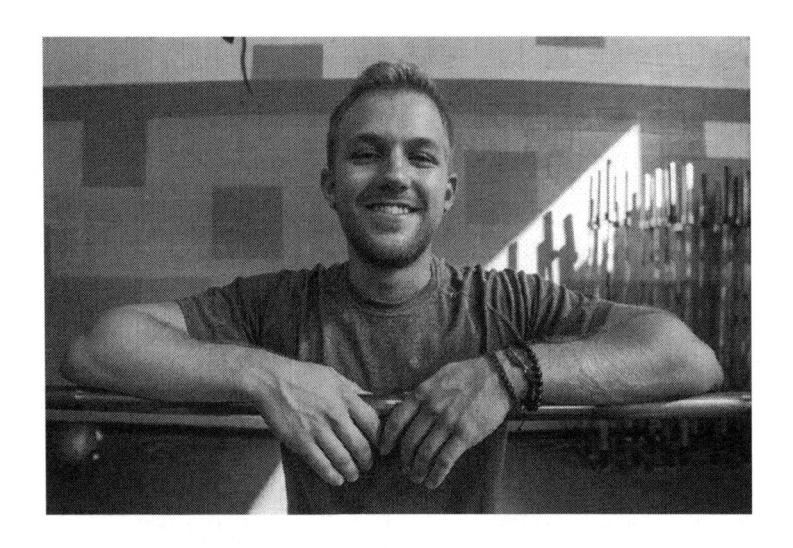

Ross Johnson is the founder of Movement Empire, an online-based fitness community that connects top coaches with students for the same reason: To pursue ability over aesthetics.

For nearly 8 years, Ross has gone into full immersion with many different physical practices, only to discover subtle cultural or dogmatic flaws in each one that prevent development. It wasn't until Ross attended trade school for personal training that he realized how much of a mess the fitness industry is.

Movement Empire is the result of his passion for wanting to help talented coaches reach more people, and expand their communities. Now, he helps fitness coaches share their best knowledge by creating digital programs that anyone can benefit from.

For more information, visit www.MovementEmpire.com.

Chapter 10: Psychology In Fitness Training

By Marcos Sayon
Alhambra, California

My career is about helping people get fit through personal training. I am from Alhambra, California, where there's an abundance of job opportunities; jobs make people busy, and busy people have no time for exercise. So, what happens? Some people grow obese and unhealthy, so suddenly they're struggling to get fit. For fifteen years, I've been telling people that they can get fit no matter how busy their office schedule is, because so much of fitness training is psychological.

I Was Once Like Them

As a kid, I used to eat a lot without minding my weight. I am Mexican, and both of my parents are Mexicans. We all know what we have in Mexico: a lot of good-tasting, enticing-smelling food. I was in high school, and then in college, when I started to gain the most weight—exactly the time when most teenagers are becoming more conscious of their appearance. Unlike a lot of others my age, I didn't care what other people thought of me. I cared only about myself, so I fed myself more often. Before I entered college, I weighed almost 175 pounds. I earned my college degree with 245. But I didn't give a damn.

Self-Awareness Is Vital

I was extremely happy with my life. I could eat whatever food I wanted, I could go out and enjoy the breeze, I could play sports, and I had Mexican parents who cook more often. I had a real zest for life, until one line hit me: "You are a fat-ass."

I really did not see it coming. I was playing basketball at the time, wearing my usual sweatshirts and shorts, never thinking I'd meet such a rude player. I was totally unprepared. But suddenly, I was also very aware of my weight.

Right then, I decided to look for a change—not to look better in the eyes of other people, but to make myself better than who I was during that game. I started thinking it was the right time to start working on a physically fit me.

Motivation and Commitment

I had friends with daily gym schedules—and I knew that they were working out to be more noticeable to girls. Since I wasn't so interested in getting the attention of the girls on our campus, I didn't really see any point in working out. I thought for that maybe I should just put the time they spent in the gym towards any other activity that could make me extremely happy.

But then I remembered that guy at the basketball court (20 years ago now). I realized that I could use that moment to motivate myself to do physical training, the same way that my friends motivated themselves with girls. I challenged myself.

From then on, I strove hard to get fit. In my first week, I started eating consciously. I counted my calorie intake and jotted down every single food I ate—after a few weeks of doing that, I could actually remember the calorie count for each type of food. I knew then that I could actually lose weight all by myself. I started gaining confidence.

Soon, I found that I finally had the guts to talk to new people. Before my commitment to fitness, I wasn't much of a talker, and I blamed shyness. I actually thought that I was introvert, until a moment came when I confronted myself about the real reason why I was sort of afraid to talk to people. Was it shyness? Or was it my weight?

I concluded that my weight had something to do with it. So, to be able to talk to more people and overcome my introversion, I explored more ways to lose more weight. I started reading books and even enrolled myself in a gym. Observing the trainers there, I noticed that the routines were actually simple; maybe I could teach them to other people.

Been There, Done That

I tried talking to people with the same problem as mine. I told them what I did, and they all tried it step by step. They told me they were improving. That was when I decided to become a trainer. After three years of work, I earned my training certificate; it's an accomplishment I'll always be proud of.

I really enjoy my job. My clients set goals, and I help them achieve those goals. I'm so passionate about helping them because I knew what it feels like, and what the possible consequences are of being overweight and unhealthy. Indeed, a lack of confidence can affect job performance, relationships with other people, and our own happiness. I am obsessed with eradicating that; I want people to be more outgoing so they can enjoy life more. *Carpe diem!*

Busy People Can Get Fit

In my fifteen years of service, most of the people I've trained have been businessmen. In my initial interviews with them, I often find that they're discouraged to go to the gym because they think it's a waste of time. They tell me that they only get extra tired, and that makes them feel more unproductive.

And I get that. But I always emphasize that they need to motivate themselves. While I understand that they need time for their work and relationships, they also need time for themselves. Hey: if I was able to do it, anyone can.

It's All In Your Mind

"Going to the gym will make me tired" is only true in your mind. You can be so productive in the gym the same way you are productive while you are in your office. You just have to internalize and embrace it.

For instance: I allot 30 minutes of my day to work out. You don't have to waste three hours waiting in a gym to be seen by a trainer. You may just need to wake up 30 minutes earlier than usual—but half an hour can be more productive than a three-hour stay in the gym if you already know what you should do, and what you want to achieve.

Heart Rate Monitoring

Heart rate monitoring makes the 30-minute workout vastly more efficient. Through this monitoring system, my clients can identify their progress: are they working slow or working fast? I believe that it is important for them to see firsthand how they are working really hard to get fit. It contributes to their drive to continue working out.

Heart Rate Monitoring is especially important for recovery. We set the 30-minute workout to avoid being burnt out. Monitoring shows that our heart gets tired as well, and so we need to rest. I use heart rate monitoring to see where my clients are already at their peak, and where they are losing their performance.

Less Trainer, More Coach

Busy people want to make the most of their day, lessening dead time like being stuck in traffic as they drive to the gym, or waiting around the gym for their fitness trainers. With those reasons, it's understandable that I've got a few clients I seldom see at the gym.

Of course, I can't keep track of my clients all the time, especially when they choose to do their training at home. But, more than a trainer, I consider myself a coach. I just don't teach training routines; I also advise clients to mind what food they eat, and the other activities that they do. From my perspective, the real fitness is not about the workout, but about the supporting programs we set for the rest of our daily habits.

I usually tell my clients that they don't need me every time they work out. They can use their equipment at home, or just surf the internet to discover new and useful routines. Part of what makes fitness training a training of oneself is that it tests our self-accountability.

My task as a trainer ends after I teach a client a new routine, but my task as a coach is endless and continuous. If a client fails to do their training today, I will ask them why. Understanding the psychology of their shortcomings shows me where I can help them improve.

Knowledge Is Power

People don't always recognize the importance of getting enough exercise because they lack knowledge. New clients often tell me that not only is no one there to motivate them, but they don't know how to go about actually working out. They know they need to get fit, but they have no idea where to start.

That is why we, fitness trainers, are here: to teach people routines, to help them turn their daily routines into healthy ones, and to motivate them to bring their brains when they exercise. It's absolutely true that physical wellness is all in your mind.

You Can Do It!

A lot of the people I used to train are now showing that their engagement with a more active lifestyle has resulted in a really positive change. From being unaware of their physical characteristics and health situations, they have built strong bodies and healthy lives. They are all saying, "I finally did it!" after years of struggle to get fit. They have changed, and it all started with one good decision.

Welcome change, and change will happen. First, be self-aware. Don't let some jerk look you head-to-toe and tell you you're a fat-ass. Second, embrace the reality that you're unhappy with your weight. Third, try to start motivating yourself. Look for the reason why you are striving to be fit: do you need other people's attention, or are you doing it for a change in yourself? Like car keys, motivation causes everything to start. But it can't come from other people, it must come from you. Motivation is part of the psychology of fitness training.

Fourth, you need to prove to yourself that you are dedicated to what you're doing. You need to be responsible not just for you, but for the people who are also rooting for your fitness. With motivation, dedication and responsibility should also be on your mind.
Finally, you need to monitor your activities to make sure you're staying on track. Then, motivate yourself to keep up the good work! When you're satisfied with the results, share your story with other people.

You can be fit even without having your whole life at a gym. You can still be productive while working on a healthier body. As I said, and as I will always say: "It is all in your mind."

Carpe diem!

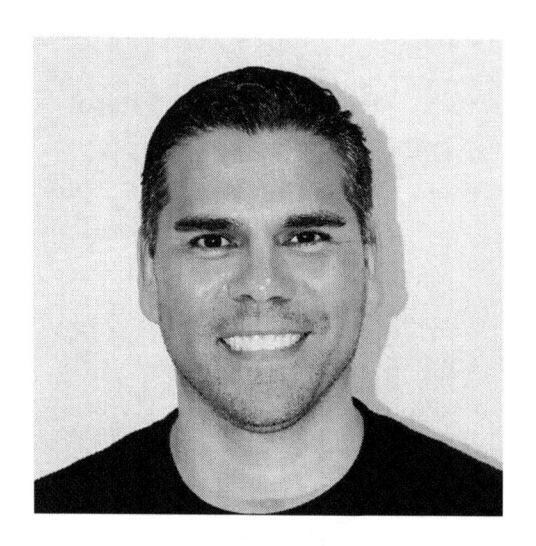

Marcos Sayon was born and raises in Southern California, a graduate of California State University of Los Angeles.

Marcos has been a Personal Trainer since 2001. He has trained thousands of clients with many fitness backgrounds, however, specializes in training for fat loss and "toning up".

A son of a migrant family. Marcos is married to his beautiful wife Maria and they have one handsome son Estevan.

For more information, visit www.sayonfit.com.

Chapter 11: Healthy Together

By Tracy Hammons
Broken Arrow, Oklahoma

When someone mentions the word "health," many of us have only ever thought about our own bodies and our own minds. "Health" is, traditionally, a very personal word. People can't be healthy for you. They can't eat for you, exercise for you, hydrate for you, or think for you. All of those things that lead to a better you must be done by you.

Protecting and taking good care of yourself should be one of the simplest biological imperatives in the world, shouldn't it? But it's harder than it seems. These days, we stress so much about the people we care about, and do so much for them, that we forget to take care of ourselves.

Thankfully, the wellbeing of our spouses, friends, and especially our children can be wonderful inspirations to take our own health seriously, and if you can make yourself healthier, that can encourage the people you love to do the same.

When embarking on any journey of change, the relationships you have with the people around you must be preserved. If not, a dangerous rift might form between the person or people trying to change and the person or people who aren't as committed. You've also heard of the importance of an accountability partner or a coach; this is the person you trust and respect who has a front-row seat to your progress and your decisions, the person you think of when that bacon double cheeseburger with grilled onions is sitting in front of you. "Do I really want to have to tell them that I ate this when we promised each other we wouldn't...?" Those are critical relationships as well, especially if they keep us from making bad choices.

As a spouse and a parent, you are in a particularly great position to be a fierce accountability partner and a good role model for every member of your family. I started working with kids as soon as I became a nurse in 1992. Even back then, my role was to help educate parents on how to help their kids live better lives and how to share that better life with them.

Education: Not Just for Kids

No one wants to make bad decisions when it comes to children, but it's so hard to make the right ones when this "go go go" lifestyle starts taking its toll on our bodies and our lives. When the kids are in bed and the workday is done, the last thing we want to do is plan meals and grocery lists, study nutrition charts, or listen to another health expert preach at us.

Still, I am a huge advocate for education, because there is such a lack of it out there for mothers and fathers and guardians in the United States. Kids may get tidbits of health trivia in school, but it's often not enough. I have watched so many wonderful families become unhealthy from the top, down.

I run a martial arts academy with my husband. Not long after we started, we noticed the shockingly sudden rise in childhood obesity—kids sitting in front of TVs and video games all day long, putting on weight, not working out, and not realizing that they need to be moving much more. The parents we talked to wanted to take care of their kids, but they didn't even know what good nutrition was. They wanted to help, but they lacked the knowledge needed to create a system that worked for their whole family.

Some parents would bring their children to martial-arts class after grabbing McDonalds or leave and immediately head off for pizza. They'd look at me apologetically or defensively and say, "We just don't have time for anything else."

There's nothing wrong with some junk food every now and then, but this was happening far too often to be the occasional guilty treat. Those same parents asked, "Why is my kid overweight, when I bring him or her to your class three times a week?"

I was led to utilize my history in medicine as well as my expertise in fitness. We created customized nutrition and exercise plans for the families in our academy to help the children become healthier. Sure enough, as the kids learned more, they started sharing the knowledge with their friends, and the parents talked to other parents, and the ripple effect continued from there.

One of the most common nutritional hang-ups I see are families trying to maintain separate diets. Maybe Mom or Dad or both are trying to feed themselves one thing in accordance to a new diet, while feeding their kids something else. Kids will duplicate what they see, not what they hear, and it's impossible to have a truly harmonious table when some people are eating salads and others are eating pizza.

As we know, the dining room table at home is only half the battle. Unfortunately, some school programs don't serve our kids' nutritional needs the way we'd like. It may be time to think about packing a healthy lunch or finding another solution.

Cafeteria pizza and fries on a daily basis can be damaging to more than just a child's body. Exposure to lots of salt and sugar as a young age can create lifelong cravings that can hinder their ability to eat well. Exposing children to lots of different healthy (and tasty!) foods as early as possible will help their minds crave what their bodies need. It's important to come up with really yummy meals and snacks that everybody in the family can enjoy, so dietary changes don't fall apart due to boring, bland options.

Starting a Routine

When a parent comes to me asking what they can do to bolster the health of their family, my first goal is to determine their commitment level. This isn't a reflection of their character or their love for their family, but for some personality types, a small change here and there is much easier than a major life overhaul. No matter what those changes are, or how small, it's an improvement upon where they were before. That's progress.

The speed, size, and style of change depends on the personality types in the entire family. Some families are ready to throw out everything in the pantry, buy a home gym for themselves, buy a membership to the local pool, and plan a hike in the mountains—all at once. Other families have individuals who would back into a corner and shut down from intimidation if you tried that.

So it's important to determine how children and families are wired before making any decisions on how to move forward with changes—large or small. For example, my kids are relatively laid back except for my youngest, who is an excited, energized go-getter. So if we sit down at a family meeting and say, "Over the next month, we're going to cut these foods out of our meals," our youngest will be instantly on board and excited to swear off of the food in question. Our other kids, who are a little resistant to change, may take more time.

When you look at the totality of health, you need to acknowledge the mental and psychological aspects of change, routine, and habit. When a sedentary person decides to be more active, it's important that they don't hear messages like, "If you don't take ten thousand steps in a week, you're doing it wrong!"

It's much better to say something simpler and much easier to achieve, like, "You need to move." That may mean taking a walk after work, riding a bike, going to an exercise class, or just taking the stairs instead of the elevator every day. For kids especially, try focusing on how long they're moving as opposed to what they're doing. If you don't want them sitting in front of the television for four or five hours a day, you can say, "Hey, you need to be up and moving right now," then let them figure out for themselves how they want to spend that time.

If you're moving, you're moving. That's all that matters.

My husband has had two hip replacements, so he is physically incapable of walking the much-acclaimed ten-thousand steps per week right now, but he has never seen that as an excuse to do nothing at all. We are constantly looking for new and creative ways to move that are enjoyable and beneficial to both of us.

Starting a new exercise or nutrition routine isn't easy for anyone, but these are some ways to make it easier. The good news is that, as a parent, you can personalize the routine in a way that doesn't make it too scary or extreme for your family. There's not just one path to true health; you can get there in a multitude of different ways that also maintains the family structure and, most importantly, keeps everyone happy and engaged.

Think Small, Achieve Big

Any self-help book can outline the parameters of wonderful diets and fitness routines that have worked for other people, but we know that every family is different and deserves its own customized system of health. It's dishonest to present any mighty, all-encompassing solution to a complex problem and claim it will work for everyone.

That being said, I have impressive anecdotal evidence that amazing things happen when a person starts examining their routines and habits and adjusts them—in a way that works for them—towards a journey of true health.

Our team has worked extensively with the mother of a wonderful four-year-old boy who has autism. He has trouble making eye-contact, is easily overwhelmed by too much sensory information, and was completely non-verbal. We suggested the mother try a certain supplement for him, and within a month, her child was speaking full sentences. Now, is this a supplement that will work with all autistic children? No. But this one mother's attempt to actively tend to the total health of her child reaped wonderful results.

Another great client we're working with right now has had Lyme disease since 2011, and all the nasty symptoms that come along with it: extreme fatigue, brain fog, achy joints, and terrible headaches. It is a truly debilitating condition that has kept her from being the person, mom, or wife she wants to be. In an eight weeks period, she's made some small changes to her diet and added a few supplements to round out her nutrition, and now, her energy level is up, her pain level is down, and she's off of 80% of her medications.

One more woman I know is bravely facing a whole host of challenges: osteoarthritis, PTSD, and menopause all at once. All of these things have created an incredible oxidative stress load on her body. Thankfully, we've figured out some ways to make her body produce tens of thousands of times her own antioxidants to help relieve this pressure. Six weeks later, her night sweats are gone. She's using her hands. She's off many of her medicines, and she's just signed up for kickboxing classes... why? Because she can!

These solutions work for these people, and I love helping them figure out a unique plan to use holistic strategies to relieve pain and stress, and to help them reduce the symptoms of truly unbearable conditions.

The Time Is Now

Eleven years ago, the New England Journal of Medicine put out the warning call when they reported that "the youth of today may, on average, live less healthy and possibly even shorter lives than their parents." That's how quickly nutrition is going downhill in this country. The Center for Disease Control (CDC) reports that "in 2012, more than one third of children and adolescents were overweight or obese". Even more stunning than the seriousness of this problem is the lack of attention people are paying to it. If you are a parent, the job of raising your child to be healthy does not fall to a teacher, or coach, or cafeteria worker, or pastor, or any other individual in your kid's life. As parents, it's our job and our honor to make sure that our children eat healthy, that they are disciplined enough to take care of themselves when we're not around, that they learn what they need to learn about health before it's too late.

They should know that the physical aspects of health include moving a lot more than they think they should and putting the right things into their body. They should know there's nothing wrong with a family movie night, but trying to find ways to be active with their loved ones is much better. They should know that the mental aspect of health is just as important: having lots of options, making changes they're comfortable with (but always seeking improvement), and strengthening their minds with new experiences that build self-esteem.

When the whole family is on board with these ideas, everything will begin to work symbiotically. When you eat better, you feel like being more active. When you feel like being more active, you'll want to spend that time with your kids or spouse. One aspect of health will inform and motivate all of the others in a positive direction. Being healthy together is better than being healthy alone.

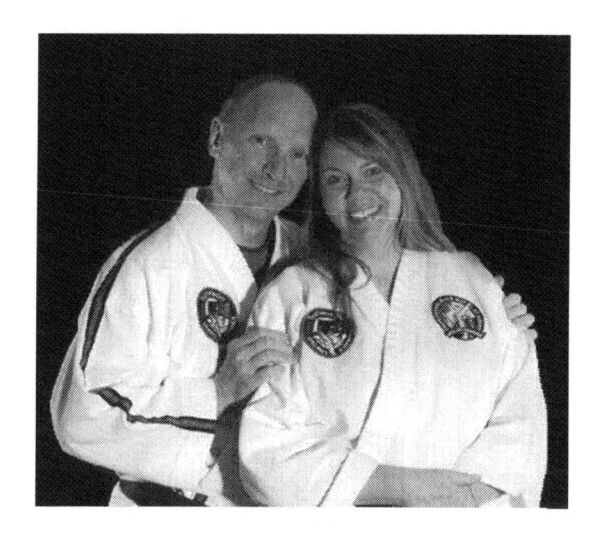

Tracy Hammons owns and operates Martial Arts Advantage in Broken Arrow, Oklahoma along with her husband Jim.

Tracy is a 1st Degree Black belt and has been training in martial arts for 16 years. She has training as a Registered Nurse and an extensive background through her martial arts instruction in working with children and families.

For more information visit www.martialartsadvantage.net.

Chapter 12: The Definition of True Health

By Gina Faubert
Burlington, Ontario, Canada

Any time the conversation comes up about how to be truly healthy, it raises the question what is health. For each of us its different, and yet poor health is very obvious. Over the past 20 years in the health industry, my own definition of True Health has evolved. My personal health & client experiences have led me to a better understanding of how to undeniably create the health we desire.

The health industry is a constant never stagnant industry bursting with new ideas in science every day. For everything you should eat, you can read a study that says you shouldn't. For every great fitness fad, there is a consequence to it's benefits. But one thing I've noticed that is a constant, and never changing, is to be consistently healthy, you have to be in the right mindset. Even those who are not in the right mindset, embarking on a fitness or nutrition programs, rarely achieve the results they desire - especially in a sustainable way.

My expansion of skills in biomechanics, physiology, and chemistry lead me to understand solid strategies for fitness program design and nutrition counseling. Studying hormones, and genes and how they can enhance our performance and body shape is a key component to many of my clients' successes. But all the knowledge of body science is ultimately not what makes the biggest impact on my clients' health. The study of Psychology - understanding why people do what they do, has paved the way to getting started, staying on track, and maintaining lasting results. I was always in search of ways to create a healthier body, but ultimately what was always a constant was the wellness from the mind. When clients succeed it was because they had unwavering commitment, enjoyment in the rituals, and a way of thinking that supported their intentions.

In each of us, we have aspirations to feel good. The steps we take each day - consciously and unconsciously are attempts to meet our needs and values. Health isn't an end goal. It's a daily practice of rituals repeated day after day, often without conscious thought to help us have that feel good feeling. Each of us has a journey of health with ebbs and flows, moving towards and away from True Health. What I've discovered is, with the right mindset we will make better decisions about our health, stay on track longer, be inspired to move and eat well, and maintain healthy rituals even when obstacles are presented. Despite my years of training, this wasn't always clear to me.

My Own Personal Journey

As a child, I lived in an environment where there were a lot of examples of people around me who were unhealthy, and suffering. I was used to moving every few years, but in grade 6 I changed schools 3 times. My mom had decided to sell everything and move to a small town on Cape Breton Island. I had to leave my real dad, my friends and extended family behind. 6 months later, the dream had unraveled, we went through another move back, and eventually she divorced my step dad. As a result of these tribulations, I became anxious, sad and angry. I began to eat and sleep a lot to distract myself from the uncertainty. I gained 25 lbs that year, a lot for a 5 foot, 12-year-old girl.

As luck would have it, a special project was given to each of us in the phys ed class at my 3rd school. We were asked to put together a 30 minute aerobics routine for our class. I still remember watching the famous 20 Minute Workouts to learn some moves, and the Richard Marks love track I used for the stretching section. This project inspired my love of fitness, and transformed my body. I noticed the more I moved, the better I felt. And the better I felt, the healthier choices I made. It wasn't long before I was waking up to work out in the mornings, biking to and from school, and dancing up a sweat with friends in the evenings.

It was a lucky coincidence that in my tween years I had discovered wise words of school counselors and how moving your body could elevate your mood, and decrease stress. As I feel in love with fitness, it became my savior. My home life was saturated in drugs and alcohol addictions, financial burdens, and new partners for both my parents. And of course, I had the challenges that most tweens face in middle school like broken hearts from silly boys, girl drama, and the pressures to fit in. When I felt anxious, angry or overwhelmed, I worked out. It became my escape. My serenity from the chaos.

At 16, my fitness began to take a back seat, and school counselors where no longer available. The pressures of studying increased, and hanging out with friends became a priority. As a result, my mood swings took me into a deep depression. I missed 90 days of class that semester. I was so depressed I couldn't get dressed for school. They say I had mono, but I knew my lack of energy and interest in life was a result of feeling helpless, overwhelmed, and incapable of making a difference for my family. I quietly contemplated suicide on a regular basis as a way out of the hopelessness. One day, as I lay on the couch lethargic, I discovered Deepak Chopra. He spoke about true health being a balance in mind, body and spirit. In order to have energy you must attain health in all of these areas. It sparked something in me, a reminder to move, to breathe, and to search out empowering minds for more answers.

I found more books on personal growth, and began to reach for empowering thoughts. These words inspired me to move forward. I continued my high school years, and started going to the gym regularly and I began to mediate. Most of this exercise, and self-reflection was done in solitude. I didn't boast, or brag. I just did it. I didn't feel good at it, nor did I feel athletic. I just knew it felt good to move my body, focus on positive thoughts, and listen to inspiring message from coaches. This kept me sane, and on track.

The last year of high school was the most challenging of all. I had grown significantly and I was butting heads with my family. I felt I had no choice but to move out, and get my own place. I decided to work hard to prove I could do it. I kept my marks up and finances above water, all while I struggled to find myself, and work through my inner battles of identity and relationships. I took up running I began listening to Tony Robbins audio programs. As I put this new knowledge into practice, I gained inner strength, improved my relationships and graduated with honors. I was then accepted at a very competitive health & wellness program at George Brown College, one that would set the stage for the rest of my future.

It was a blessing that I fell into fitness at an early age. The support of amazing coaches and counselors was essential. And to be exposed to brilliant personal growth leaders was transformational. Without these resources, the deck would have been stacked against me. It's because of this that I feel so compelled to help young girls to experience movement and mindset to lay the foundation for a lifetime of True Health.

Obsessed for Results

After graduation, I began my professional career a personal trainer, and over the years, as an avid learner, I incorporated Pilates and yoga into my practice, and then added advanced nutrition education to my skills.

My focus was initially on sports performance as I worked with Canadian Olympic athletes, training our top youth to achieve incredible results. I inadvertently peppered my sessions with motivational quotes that had inspired me. I then accepted a contract training executives and a large financial institution. And that's when my eyes where opened. You see, Olympic athletes where already in a great mindset. They had a goal, they were dedicated, and excited to work hard. My inspirational words, helped them take it to the next level. My programs where easy to adhere to and reaped great results. However, my CEO's where stressed, limited schedules, big demands, and had been out of shape for years. My "perfect" Olympic programs where useless. And at first I blamed them. If only they would follow my plans they would be in great shape. In my frustration, the light bulb went on. Those who succeed are first in the right mindset. They followed through with plan with eagerness and ease.

This is what sparked my obsession with the psychology of health. I began to wonder what that mindset was that created motivation, follow through, and achievement, and the mindset that lead to struggle, self-sabotage, and quitting. I knew I had experienced it, and if I could discover the distinctions, I would be able to influence all those with good intentions to take the leap, use their mind to stay motivated, and follow through with the process. If that was possible, all my clients would achieve their goals. I became obsessed. I began to eat, sleep and breathe this vision.

I began studying everything I could find on personal growth, sports psychology, and motivation, I undertook a 2 year coaching program, and became a self-proclaimed seminar junkie. As I began applying these skills, I had more and more success with clients, and began to recognize mindset was really the root of all success in fitness.

I Knew This Stuff

A few years later, I found myself struggling to find my own True Health. I had completed my coaching certification and was running a successful personal training & coaching practice out of my wellness retreat. I had a team of health professionals, a 4-year old daughter, significant financial burdens, and my mother-in-law who came to live with us.

The stress of the situation began to take its toll on my body. Even though I was teaching classes every day, and eating well, I began to gain weight and lose energy. My mood was often less than cheerful, and in the process I developed chronic hives. I wasn't able to maintain the wellbeing I had known and lived.

I started seeking advice from others who were well versed in health, and hearing all the things I knew I should be doing. At first, I had excuses for why I wasn't doing these things. Eventually it hit me... I asked myself, "If I know all of these things—why am I not doing them?" The answer was right in front of me: the stresses in my life were affecting my health, and they'd become so overwhelming that I couldn't overcome their influences on my mind and body.

The realization that my mind was at the core of my health, lead me to dig deeper into psychology. I began studying neuro-linguistic programming (NLP) and mental-emotional release therapy, both strategies developed by some of the world's leading therapists. Essentially, they are tools and techniques that uncover deep issues, typically in the subconscious mind, in a short amount of time. Some of the best coaches and therapists in the world use these techniques, and are able to see significant results sometimes within a single session. They're incredibly powerful strategies that reveal underlying mental blocks, effecting shifts and changes in people on a much deeper level than just positive self-talk. The results where incredible for me. I was able to overcome my health challenges, and return back to a strong healthy state. And my coaching sessions have never been the same since.

What You Believe You Will Achieve

Today, I use all these tools in my health coaching sessions to help adults and children create True Health. We begin with an overview of what's really going on in their lives. I listen for what inspires them, what holds them back, and their strategies for dealing with stress. Our bodies are designed to move, and we feel good when we eat right, so when we don't, we are meeting our needs in unproductive ways. If we can get to the root of core issues, and create new empowering ways to meet our needs, these self-sabotaging behaviors fall away, and health plans are easily followed.

One of my favorite tools is called the Wheel of Life. I ask clients to rate each category of their life from 1-10. Categories like health, career, finances and spouse for adults, and for kids categories like school, friends, and hobbies. Then I ask them what would make each of these categories a 10/10. This creates a clear vision of the life they desire. Next, I ask them why isn't it that way now. And this determines the limiting believes, stresses, and patterns of behavior that prevent them from living their best. Anyone at any age can create a wheel of life plan.

Once we have determined their vision and limitations, we go to work on making both. A clear vision for what you want to create allows you to see opportunities, make decisions easily, and effortlessly follow through with intentions. We spend time describing the pictures and emotions we expect to have in these categories. With my girls' programs we make dream boards to look at daily and remind us of our intentions. With adults the vision may take the form of a daily mediation practice, or journal writing. Positive visualization is great, but without addressing the limitations it loses its energy, and intentions are stalled or sidetracked by the stresses of life.

The most important part of the work I do, is helping people overcome their mental blocks. Mental blocks that limit you from achieving your goals are called limiting beliefs, and they are often hard to spot on oneself. These mental blocks prevent us from getting to our workouts, eating how we intended, or following through with mediation. These blocks are a big part of our unconscious mind, and even when we shed light on limiting beliefs, and disempowering patterns, they can't be changed consciously. Willpower can't overcome beliefs. This is the reason self-sabotage returns. In addressing these blocks with coaching techniques like anchoring, swish patterns, mapping across and mental emotional release, we can affect the unconscious mind and make significant changes to the root causes, which is what creates results.

To find out what your limiting beliefs are, ask yourself "What am I most stressed about?"
Although everyone has different circumstances, the root cause of most stress for both adults and kids is 1. Fear of not being loved, 2. Fear of not being enough, 3. Loss of Happiness. The good news is, these limiting beliefs can be overcome.

What You Value You Do

Another common reasons for procrastination is that the goals are not in line with one's values. For example, I often hear there's not enough time. I understand that time is limited, and finding time can be extraordinarily difficult for many of us, but the question of time is more a question of value than anything else. You have to ask yourself what's most important in your life - what do you value, and from there you allocate your time accordingly. And, as we look back, we evaluate our time based on what we value. If you value spending time with your kids, making a difference in the world, and feeling successful and your workouts where spent in isolation, focused on yourself, and too difficult to complete, you will be unlikely to continue. When I discover what a person's values are, we can then design a health program that fits these values, so their goals and intentions are congruent.

As a parent one of the most valuable things we can do for our kids is create a list of values and beliefs we'd like them to adopt. Once this list has been established, we can review the list regularly, and we can teach these values on a consistent basis. When we tell stories, give reasons for our decisions, or discipline our kids, we have a foundation of empowering principles that we are basing these actions on. Imagine how powerful it could be for a parent to instill in a child the value of taking care of your body and mind, and then reaffirm it throughout the formative years. As a result, there is a high probability these values will extend into their adult with ease.

Setting the Stage for Success

Now that I know better, I take a different approach when I start working with both adults and kids. Before I begin on the perfect workout and nutrition plan that's best for their body, I begin with their mind. I ask them to paint me a picture of what True Health really means to them. Next we determine all the reasons that have prevented them from taking better care of their body. And then we determine the strategies they use to deal with stress and challenges.

With this clarity, I help clients release limiting patterns & beliefs, create new empowering strategies to overcome challenges, and then a solid fitness & nutrition plan in line with their values and needs. This method creates an energy and a desire to succeed because we've gone further than "Do this because it's the right thing" It's not a one-size-fits-all program, it's a program designed on what makes you tick. This holistic view enables us to a create a transformation plan that becomes a consistent enjoyable part of your lifestyle. With the right resources, anything is possible.

Embarking on your Health Journey

Before you begin signing a gym contract, or starting a new diet plan, consider setting your mind up for success first. Create a vision for what it YOUR True Health. What does it mean to you to be your Personal Best? What do you really want to create?

What do you value, and how can you incorporate that into your goals? What fitness or nutrition plan will allow you to meet your values each and every time?

Ask yourself what has stopped you in the past, what may stop you this time? Seek out a coach, or trainer who can help you overcome those possible obstacles with solid support. Someone with NLP training is best!

Best Life for Everyone

Because of the impact of fitness on my youth, I'm dedicated to inspire others to feel good with fitness, to give them strategies to escape in healthy ways, and to create positive and productive thoughts that move them towards their best life. My childhood did have a number of coincidences, and perfect situations that inspired me to be my best, despite the conditions. I feel it was my destiny so that i could be the catalyst for kid and teens to discover the benefits of movement and mindset.

I'm equally as motivated to share my coaching strategies with adults who are on the path of discovering their Best Life. The truth is that anyone and everyone can get started on the path to a healthier life; it just takes a first step. When you realize that the reason you're putting off your journey to true health is just a mental block, you've gotten started. Making the decision to make a change now, is the second step. Third - take action. A single action today can be the most powerful thing you can do for your health! I know you can overcome your limitations and become excited about setting and achieving health goals, but it's up to you to take that all-important first step. Once you take it, you'll soon be on your way to achieving your own definition of True Health and living your Best Life!

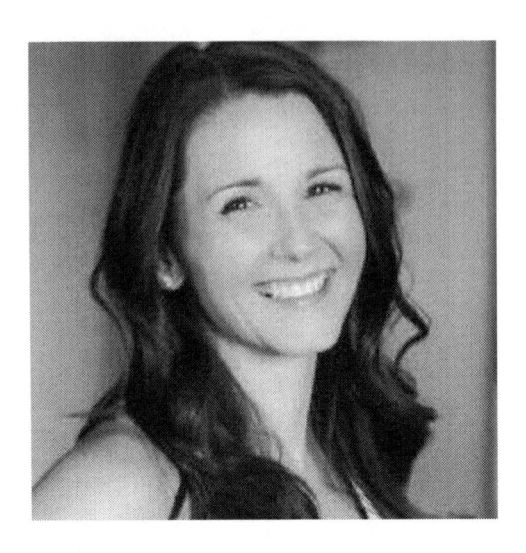

Gina's extensive expertise in fitness & lifestyle coaching started over 20 years ago when she became determined to discover how to really inspire change for great health. Her on-going quest has led her to become a certified Personal Trainer, Trained Pilates Teacher, Certified Yoga teacher, Certified Life Coach, a Master Practitioner of NLP, MER and Hypnotherapy, a BioSignature Practitioner, and holds certifications in healing modalities like Thai massage, Reiki and Reflexology. Through her years of training and speaking to Olympic athletes, Fortune 500 companies, and small business owners, she's created a system for results driven programs, life changing events and inspiring workshops.

Gina has a reputation of being a catalyst that inspires people to undergo significant shifts in their life and finally achieve their health goals. Her recommendations are backed by the latest research and proven strategies for change. She is constantly on the forefront of industry knowledge and goes to great lengths to study with the best health and fitness professionals in the world such as Tony Robbins, Charles Poliquin, Seane Corn, Dr. Natasha Turner, and Louise Hay to name a few.

She speaks regularly on the link between the mental/emotional connection to fitness, no nonsense nutrition, and developing the rituals to create exceptional health. She has soft spot for teaching girls these important lessons through camps and school seminars.

Gina holds memberships with ACMS, IFPM, ICF, BioSig, and sits on the advisory board for George Brown College's Fitness & Lifestyle Management program.

Today, Gina is available for Private Sessions, Group Classes & Workshops, Girls Camps, Wellness Retreats and Corporate Events throughout Halton & Hamilton.

Chapter 13: Qigong – Cultivating Life Energy

By Julie Balderrama
Dripping Spring, Texas

True health is a topic gaining ground in the health, wellness, and fitness industries. We naturally yearn to live the best life we can. We want to avoid illnesses associated with poor eating habits, lack of movement, and too much stress.

Discussions surrounding diet, activity, and nutrition are not only informative but also self-awakening. As an Embodied Wellness Coach and practitioner at HeartMind Healing Arts, I've worked with people using both conventional and alternative or complimentary methods to help my clients achieve desirable and, most importantly, lasting results. In addition, the tools we employ are designed to provide a solid foundation of practice that they can use whether they are at the peak of health or in the midst of devastating illness or injury - and everything in between. Times of transition in people's lives are usually the spaces where they face challenges to their health routines. It's in exactly those moments when they most need a practice like Qigong, an ancient Chinese healing modality.

What Is Qigong?

While the method may sound quite different, the Chinese healing modality called Qigong has been in use for thousands of years. Though these exercises were traditionally referred to as Dao Yin (leading and guiding the Qi), the word Qigong came to be used to describe this art in the mid 20th century. Qi, in Chinese means "life force energy." Gong means to "cultivate" or "refine." So Qigong is the practice of developing and refining one's personal life energy. This is a Body, Mind, Heart, and Spirit practice with healing potential available at every level and stage of a person's life.

Does Cultivating Life Energy Help Achieve True Health?

Absolutely! The best thing about Qigong is its availability. You don't have to have any special equipment or specific place to practice. You can be in any physical condition - and I do mean any (Qigong is often used in hospitals as a compliment to other healing modalities). And it can be completely free!

Qigong is an excellent way to prevent and heal disease, relieve pain, and improve overall physical health. And unlike other medical interventions, Qigong has no side effects! This slow, gentle, and mindful practice allows you to immerse into the parasympathetic state (sometimes called "rest and digest") which is where the body heals. It's the opposite of our sympathetic state in our nervous system - or fight or flight. When you're in this relaxed space, it honestly doesn't matter much how much you engage physically, as long as you practice intentionally, with your mind in the present moment.

We know that somewhere around 80% of preventable disease is caused by stress - by chronically occupying the sympathetic part of the nervous system. Spending anywhere between 5 minutes to an hour or more a day in this relaxed state goes a long way to reducing the number of preventable diseases.

Of course True Health is about more than our body. To achieve True Health, we want to also pay attention to our mind, our emotions, and our spirit. When we take exquisite care of our body, mind, heart, and soul, we have True Health. Qigong gives us the ability to do exactly that.

Personal

Qigong is a Body Mind practice, so it can transcend physical healing in the body. Some practitioners experience relief from suffering with everything from grief to anxiety and depression. Anger and frustration or stress can also feel more manageable with this internal practice.

Along with many of my clients and students, I've personally found deep healing from emotional suffering through Qigong. After my daughter was born, I was in a dark space emotionally. My physical body was foreign to me and I felt isolated and depressed. I didn't know who I was anymore. But I did know that I had a child to care for. Qigong helped me back to myself so I could be the mother I wanted to be. It changed my life. And I've seen it change so many other lives as well.

Qigong can be what we refer to as an Alchemical practice, meaning that we start with the raw materials of the physical body and through disciplined cultivation of our internal energy, we heal any emotional dis-ease so we can then reveal our true divine selves. What's amazing about this process is that it isn't necessarily linear. You might experience your true divine self while your body or heart is still suffering. But touching the divine makes that suffering just a bit more bearable. In fact, getting in touch with this part of ourselves is the shift that makes loving kindness and conscious choice possible.

The truth is: You are Awesome exactly as you are. You aren't broken, there's nothing wrong with you. You don't need to be fixed. You are eternally well and whole. It is through Qigong that we can find the part of ourselves that knows and remembers this - no matter what our physical body looks or feels like, no matter how much suffering we may endure.

Is Qigong Different From Tai Chi?

The main difference between Qigong and Tai Chi is that Qigong is more of an Internal Practice, while Tai Chi is a balance between internal and external practice. Some refer to Qigong as the Mother of Tai Chi. I would say this is true both historically and from the perspective of the natural flow of energy through the practices. Tai Chi, to be effective, must have a foundation of Qigong. Both practices play with Yin and Yang energy as a means of personal cultivation. Yin and Yang are the two energies that makeup the entire Universe.

If you think of a vertical line, Yin would be on the left side; Yang, the right. Yin, is regarded as the more internal or still aspect, and Yang, the external or movement aspect. The balance of those two energies is actually called Tai Chi. So Tai Chi is the concept of supreme balance of yin and yang, which happens to have a form of martial arts named for it. Thus, Tai Chi would fall in the the middle of our Yin/Yang spectrum. Seated meditation would fall all the way on the Yin or still side. Kung Fu would land all the way to the right - a very Yang and external practice.

Qigong is mostly an internal practice with some gentle external movements, which usually repeat, offering a more meditative quality to the movements. Qigong also includes four "baskets" of practice available to the student. In addition to the gentle movement, we also have self-applied acupressure, breathing techniques, and meditation practices.

Since Tai Chi is more of a balance between Yin and Yang, or internal and external, the movements can sometimes be more complex, with different sides of the body moving in different directions. These movements, which also often cross the mid-line of the body engage the brain function in a unique way that makes Tai Chi a fantastic practice for brain health. Several medical articles have praised Tai Chi as the best kind of exercise to do to ward off dementia and Alzheimer's.

The Benefits of an Internal Practice

In contemporary living, you might find a higher level of emphasis on the need to keep fit and adhere to popular diets. Most of these programs seem to be focused on achieving wellness through changing external factors: how you eat or how you move your body. Using Qigong in my wellness coaching private practice and group programs helps my clients embrace internal focus as a means to create the change they seek. We work on internal energy training by creating awareness of the state of one's Qi, or life force energy and then working with the natural flow of the energy. Your Qi is naturally tending toward health and wellness. You just have to tune in to the flow. In this way, we can make lasting, sustainable changes that are truly in the highest good for my clients.

I came to Qigong when I first tried to lose weight. I found an exercise program that worked for me, counted calories and lost some weight. But when I got to the plateau, I mistakenly believed I had to either dig in or give in to discouragement. Only after adopting Qigong did I move through that plateau to my end goal. The internal practice not only liberated me from the discouraging negative self-talk that threatened to make me give up on my goals, but it also helped me change some of my patterned behaviors that were sabotaging my success. These patterns were based on unconscious beliefs. Qigong helped me bring those beliefs into my awareness so I could shift my thoughts and my behavior.

Before Qigong, I was still operating from a place of unconscious choice. I went to the gym and did the exercises because that was what I thought I was supposed to do. I ate or didn't eat certain things because this was the path to losing weight. What I wasn't dealing with was the internal beliefs about my own inherent worthiness. Once I had a practice to address that, I could take care of my body from a very loving place. This shift made everything so much easier!

Imagine moving your body because you love it, because you want to take care of it - not because you hate it or want to punish it for not looking a certain way. Huge shift! In fact, I don't call myself a Wellness Coach, I say I'm a Self-Love Coach. When we approach life from a Loving Place, from a place of deep knowing (which you can access through Qigong) we can create remarkable, successful and sustainable progress.

Is Qigong Suitable for Seniors?

As we age, we can find ourselves with different limitations in our bodies than we're accustomed to. The activities available to us we for exercise are simply no longer accessible. Qigong is perfect for an aging population, for the healing benefits as well as preventative medicine. If you don't move it, you lose it! The good news is, you can move gently and benefit just as much as if you move more vigorously. As a coach, I've used Qigong with older adults since the practice is gentle and suitable for anybody. In fact, Qigong is perfect for seniors as it's one of the best exercises for joint health, flexibility, and maintaining balance.

Of course, anyone can be subject to illness or injury and Qigong is one of the best practices to help the body recover. I have a student who fell from his roof, fracturing his skull and dozens of other bones in his body. He recovered fully from the fall using Qigong. His doctors are still amazed! I've had students recover from knee surgery, hip surgery, and a brain tumor. I've also had students with Parkinson's see great improvement in their condition using these practices.

Qigong isn't just for an older or impaired population. Top athletes can also benefit from the practice. Not only can the gentle movements and self-applied acupressure support the body as it trains in a "harder" discipline, but the breathing techniques and meditation help the athlete with the "mind" part of their game. Meditation and visualization techniques are often a key part of an athlete's training. Qigong is simply a more external extension of this exercise. I have a student who swears that Qigong improves his golf game!

Going By the Basics

One of the things I love about Qigong is that you can do it anywhere! You don't need special equipment or clothing - or even to be in a certain kind of space. You can even do Qigong when you're driving - I do it all the time! It is said that every deep breath is Qigong. In fact a simple Qigong practice is called The Remembering Breath. It goes like this: Pause for a moment and be still. Remember that you have the ability, right now, in this moment to take a deep, full breath. Then, do that. Take a conscious breath. Then another. Begin to slow your exhale and allow the fullness of your inhale. That's it! You've just done Qigong!

The breath work in Qigong is designed to move you into the parasympathetic state - where the body heals. Not only can the physical body heal, but it can also release trauma and ease emotional suffering. Very often, practitioners find a sense of inner peace or even make a profound connection with their Higher Power.

Connecting to our true sense of self can effect behavioral change too since calm, well-centered people can consciously respond to situations, instead of reacting out of habit or with heightened emotions.

The Remembering Breath - and any practice that helps you make conscious choices can help you change your habits or your behavior. The brain forms a habit loop with a cue, the action, and a reward. Undoing that loop or forming a new loop requires the ability to put some space between the cue and the action - so you can perform a different action - in order to be successful. A simple breath and return to the present moment can be a big help in that process.

Imagine that you're sitting down to watch TV at night. You usually have a little snack in your hands as you're watching. But you've decided that you no longer want to snack at night. The cue is sitting down to watch TV. The action is eating a snack. Taking just a moment or a breath to remember that you don't want a snack can be the thing that unwires this habit loop.

This works for our reactions in stressful situations too. When someone expresses displeasure with me, my habit is to get defensive and sometimes angry. But I would rather respond by listening to what they have to say - letting go of what doesn't feel true and adjusting my behavior (and perhaps apologizing) where appropriate. To respond this way, I have to have some space between the cue and the action to remember what I want.

David Campbell said, "discipline is remembering what you want." The Remembering Breath helps you remember what you want (and what you don't want!).

How Long Does It Take to Practice?

You can practice 5 minutes a day and see results. Of course, the more you practice, the better the results. My teacher says "It's better to do it wrong than not at all." You'll read books that tell you to practice for an hour a day. Or to only practice in the morning. Or only practice on an empty stomach. None of that should hold you back.

Just practice. Whatever you can. For however long you can.

While most people will see results fairly soon after starting Qigong, we all vary in our ability to grasp and master any modality. How well a person will respond to Qigong depends largely on if they're willing to try - just for a moment - to quiet the internal voices. If you can get into that parasympathetic state by staying relaxed and breathing deeply, you'll feel good by the end of your first class. It might take a few more classes, but with enthusiastic curiosity, you'll get there!

The Key to a Great Program

First, find a practice that resonates with you. If you don't immediately find a teacher who suits your style, try a few other instructors and forms. There are so many different styles of

Qigong and so many different types of teachers. If you don't enjoy a class or it doesn't seem to be helping you, seek out a different teacher until you find one you like.

Secondly, I recommend teachers who give some level of autonomy and self-empowerment, instead of those who insist on a certain way of doing things. I think one of the reasons I embraced Qigong so enthusiastically was because of my own teacher, Dr. Roger Jahnke, O.M.D. (his book, The Healer Within is a great resource for starting your Qigong practice!). Dr. Jahnke always tells us: Let the Practice be the Master.

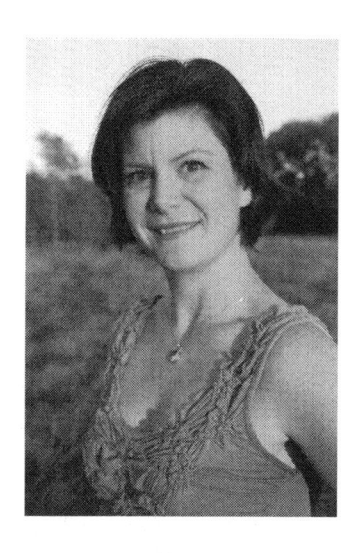

Julie Balderrama is a Self-Love Coach and certified Qigong teacher. She's passionate about empowering her clients, students, and followers to live a life with purpose and conscious choice. Through Qigong practices and coaching techniques she guides people in turning pain into pleasure, critical self-talk into loving presence, and harmful habits into a radical Self Love Practice.

For more information, visit www.heartmindqi.com.

Chapter 14: Health, Wealth, and Happiness

By Alex Klaus
Charlotte, North Carolina

In modern Western society, we are obsessed with surrounding and filling ourselves with dangerous, work-centric ideologies. We fuel notions of "hustling" and "making it." We work our way up impressive ladders and buy just the right material possessions to prove we've done it. We say things like, "I can sleep later" and shamelessly glorify 60- to 80-hour work-weeks.

I spent far too many years of my life trying to fit this "success" script—buying into, complying with, and even rebelling against outside notions of what my life was supposed to be as a business developer and strategist.

Mentally, I focused intensely on my goals, acquiring strategic and tactical business knowledge. I frantically expanded my network, building million-dollar businesses with several more in the pipeline.

Emotionally, I was obsessed with creating a life without financial failure, which I realized later had been my worst fear the entire time.

Physically, I slowly but surely deteriorated from my former athletic teen self, gained weight, and drew on the physical capacity I had built in the decades prior. But even that seemed a small price to pay for achieving my (and society's) goal of "making it."

I've always had, I believe, the best of intentions, a big heart for people, and an intensely hopeful drive, but I spent many years focused on a financial status I wanted but that did not come from my core. Certain events helped me discover that financial success was just *one* key to happiness, not the *only* key.

It all started with a business investment that I miscalculated in many ways. First, it cost me about $150,000 more than I had intended. Some of that money wasn't mine, which was a huge source of guilt for me. The venture did not become cash-flow positive for a lot longer than I had projected, and the long-term lack of sleep, overworking, and pulling myself out of nurturing relationships in order to pour myself into the business caused me to burn out in months.

Because I placed such a high value on being financially stable, it felt as though being financially instable was more than just a failure—it was a threat to my very existence.

Ironically, I was soon after awarded "Distinguished Alumnus of the Year" by my alma mater, Coastal Carolina University, as the youngest ever and first international student to receive this once-in-a-lifetime honor. However, the joy of the occasion felt confusing in light of my great failure, and evaporated quickly. The one thing I was good at—business—started to interest me less and less. What would become of me?

The exhaustion led to several mental distortions, which today I call my "bullshit stories." First, that my self-worth depended on economic outcomes, and second, that a failure to achieve a financial goal meant that I was a failure as a person. With enough sleep and awareness, these would have been considerably different stories from the start—I would've been able to look at that $150,000 and say, "It's just money!"—but my work habits and work attitudes were based on a "live-to-work" mentality that is very widespread today.

Eventually I discovered that the fledgling business just needed more time and money to become financially viable. It was far from being a failure. In fact, it's still open and thriving

These days, I believe there really is no such thing as a "failure" if you learn something from the experience... and I learned quite a bit during this particular struggle. If being in business had the power to sap the joy and happiness out of my life, perhaps it wasn't the right field for me.

Or, more likely, maybe I was approaching business as though I had to conform to its needs and desires, rather than letting it conform to mine.

It's All In Your Head

I've always been the type of person to accept full responsibility for my life, for the outcomes I create and all of the actions that got me there. Perhaps that's why looking at myself in hindsight gives me such a good idea of the person I was versus the person I knew I wanted to become.

I took a step back and looked at my life as it was, and the fogs of "success" and "failure" cleared, allowing me to see the immense chasms of emptiness in so many neglected areas of my life.

Now, I am aware of six different realms of health that must be actively nurtured: my spiritual health, my mental and emotional health, my physical health, my relationships, my professional work, and my financial health, in order of importance.

Simple changes in my routine designed to tend these areas soon became important habits: a complete night's sleep every night, limiting screen time, meditating daily, journaling, working out regularly, and connecting with family and friends. I became a vegetarian and ate an alkaline diet. Little by little, these simple things started having a profound effect. I lost 25 pounds, and my energy level soared. I have more strength and flexibility now than I did for over a decade, and my alertness and calmness enables me to retain information quicker and easier.

More important than the surface-level changes were the powerful shifts in perception I underwent. We all have those "bullshit stories" holding us back, and breaking through mine opened a Pandora's box of possibilities that I could never have imagined.

These days, I define "Wealth" as small efforts producing big outcomes, or small actions that allow us to show up fully charged in all areas of life. For me, it's getting a complete night's sleep, making time to meditate or journal daily, frequently connecting with family and friends, and giving myself time to let my creativity flow. Wealth is a filter I use to allocate the limited resources I have, especially time and energy.

"Inner Peace" is another filter I use to be at peace with the here and now, to trust in the path, to trust I am guided, to act from the soul, and allow myself to fully experience any emotions that make life worth living in the here and now, rather than waiting for some milestone or grand achievement to allow myself to feel happy or accomplished. (This was an important filter for a guy like me, who lived under the oppression of perfectionist tendencies for many years.)

The "Living In" filter enables emotional and physical immersion in the first two. It allows me to embody the first two filters, to make decisions and follow through with Wealth and Inner Peace in mind. If True Health were only Wealth and Inner Peace, both of them would be externalized concepts to strive for, rather than concepts to decide for, to make happen, and fully become.

The struggle I encountered in my thirties was a blessing, a gift of grace. Without it, I wouldn't feel free to take vacations to see our magnificent world, and I wouldn't be a part of a movement for a higher quality of life while enjoying the best parts of business success simultaneously. I may still be working 24/7, with parts of my family life flying by without me stopping and fully relishing them. I'd have less joy, laughter, and connection with other people.

And for what? A heart attack and a full bank account? No thank you.

When Failure is the Greatest Gift

My journey took me from building and honing business acumen, to the successful implementation of building two million-dollar businesses, to hitting a self-inflicted wall, falling down and trying to get back up, to becoming aware and eventually learning about my several own internally created walls that I have limited myself with. Now, my True Health grows in the soil of those valuable experiences and expertise.

For better or for worse, I had been entrusted with the gift of mastering business strategies. I was committed to making sure that my extensive knowledge—paid for by so many hours of blood, sweat, tears, and sleeplessness—wasn't going to go to waste. I wanted to use my years of struggle for the greater good.

Now, any business or individuals I work with have to meet a simple criteria: they must be positively and sustainably impacting human lives. The businesses I currently own or oversee provide about 30,000 massages and 100,000 chiropractic adjustments a year, and growing.

Because I'm a creative artist at heart—combined with my finance and strategy background—I now allocate time to mentor, consult, and sometimes partner with artists whose service or product meets that criteria. I truly enjoy the process of helping people overcome the mental barriers they don't know they have, and watching their lives improve as a result. I always enjoy coaching clients as my time allows.

About a year ago, I analyzed a business model pro bono, because I saw the tremendous potential it had to positively impact human lives. The company understood itself as a distributor of specialty equipment, generating income by making a one-time sale and offering very limited service. My analysis concluded that they had the opportunity to develop, from their existing core, a first-mover franchise business model that would create at least seven different streams of income, and a great opportunity to grow their existing market ten times over with sustainable, structured growth. I developed an entire blueprint for the franchise future of the company. The venture is now using the blueprint to grow a service via franchise model in the United States that will ultimately positively and sustainably impact many, many lives.

I also coached a young executive who was content and secure in his financial services job, but who was interested in following a dream that was much more rewarding but far less certain. We assessed his situation, his motives, and all of the related emotions, and over time were able to make him not just more receptive to uncertainty, but even joyful about it. Together, we built a strategic plan through several sessions that helped him create a thriving start-up. Now, he is living his dream—and my criteria—of positively and sustainably impacting people every day.

Consistency is the Key to True Health

Whenever I work with clients, there's always an introductory first conversation to assess personal fit and the client's desired outcomes. One part of that conversation is for me to better understand my potential client's attitude about consistency and commitment.

I want them to get results as fast as possible but to be committed to stay as long as necessary to see their outcome implemented and lived habitually. The one common theme I have seen in all our businesses is that people often over-estimate what they can accomplish in the short-term, and underestimate what they can accomplish in the long-term. Whether it's professional massage therapy, chiropractic care, business consulting, or my coaching clients, there's usually a total disregard of consistency.

Many clients carry the "quick fix" mindset and overlook the physical, emotional and mental benefits of making therapeutic services or coaching a regular commitment. Study after study shows the physical and emotional long-term benefits of regular massage therapy, but many clients still have to be educated, convinced, reminded and pre-scheduled to come in regularly. It's the same for people needing chiropractic care—they're in it just for the cure, not for a continuous and preventative service that improves overall health gradually, re-trains the muscles attached to the spine, and can actually result in a much-improved posture over the course of several months.

A good coach or consultant can create a shift in perspective pretty quickly, but a great coach helps you fully implement new knowledge with new decisions and new actions in life and business. This takes some time and frequency and results in new or upgraded habits, in one's life or in an organization. Some changes of perception are simply strategic or tactical, while other shifts in perception are based on overcoming personal, or internal, limiting paradigms. In a more tangible way in our operating businesses, we have built communication protocols that introduce and inform new clients of the benefits of regular care, and remind existing clients of the same at regular intervals.

It's only a challenge if we call it a challenge. Otherwise, it's an opportunity to help us differentiate ourselves in the market.

Consistency is the key to attaining any kind of success, and consistency is all to do with psychology. As a species, humans seem to act irrationally in the face of rational choices. We consume too much ice cream and not enough raw food, too many sodas and not enough water, too many hours of TV and not nearly enough time with loved ones. What is it driving our actions? If we want those actions to change, and *stay* changed, what kind of psychological leverage do we need?

I still learn daily to become even more aware of my six key areas in life. I am constantly learning and unlearning, substituting old ways, deciding on new ways, and executing those decisions. True Health is less of a mastery and more of a guiding concept in life. It never stops challenging me. It's not easy to do, but it's worth it to consciously unlearn those old habits, attitudes, values, and internal rules that no longer serve you. Substitute them with values, rules, attitudes and habits that fully support who you seek to become—spiritually, mentally, emotionally, physically, socially, professionally, and financially.

The devastatingly work-centric culture of the United States is slowly, but surely, experiencing a paradigm shift towards True Health. It will take as many people as we can get to see it through to the other side, and I am very excited to see where it will lead us.

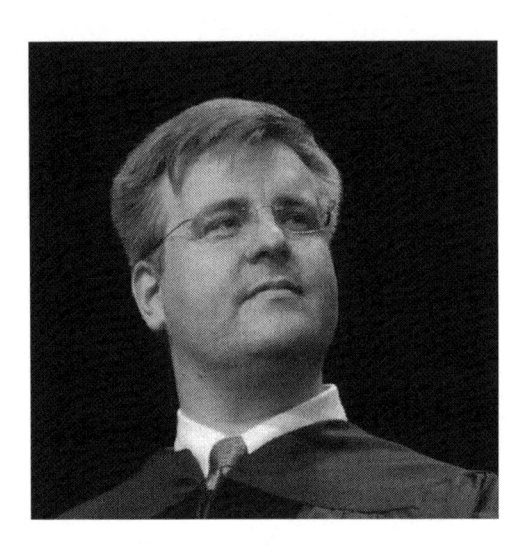

Alexander Klaus is a perpetual student. He studies business models, durable competitive advantages and psychology.

After graduating from Coastal Carolina University with a BSc in Finance and Business Administration, Alexander worked as a financial analyst for Chanticleer Holdings, Inc and avidly studied Warren Buffet, Benjamin Graham, Edward Lampert and related writings.

In 2008, he became an entrepreneur and started up a massage clinic business in Columbia, SC, where 60+ employees currently provide more than 30,000 hours of massage therapy per month to the Columbia community.

In 2011, Alexander decided to go back to the intellectually more satisfying challenge of investing, and modeled Addisco Value Partner Fund, L.P. after the original Warren Buffett partnership of 1962 with no management fee and personal funds invested alongside limited partners. In 2013, the franchise operations grew as we became Regional Developers of "The Joint...the chiropractic place" for the state of Virginia, with 19 sold licenses and 10 stores in operation.

Alexander's greatest business strength lies in focusing on durable competitive advantages, and using company-specific insight developed over time for lower risk investment decisions when opportunities present themselves.

Alexander lives in Charlotte, NC with his amazing wife Anne and their princess daughter.

Your Next Step: Decision and Action

One of my favorite quotations from Anthony Robbins is the following:

"It is in our moments of decision that our destiny is shaped."

And what a powerful quotation that is. The roots of the word "decision" mean "to cut off." This says that when you or I make a decision about something, we cut off all other options.

After reading this book, or the chapters you read, what decision are *you* going to make about living your Best Life?

Are you going to look at your environment? Your nutrition? Are you going to monitor your thoughts?

Maybe hire a professional or a mentor to help you?

Or something else?

Not only is making the *decision* important, but taking the *follow-up actions* is really what will make the difference in your life, and achieving true health in order to live the best life.

Our decisions shape our destiny. Our actions sculpt our lives.

Go out there and make magic happen for you and our world.

Made in the USA
San Bernardino, CA
31 December 2016